ESCAPE FROM MOSS PARK MENTAL HOSPITAL

a true story by
Paul Philip Studer

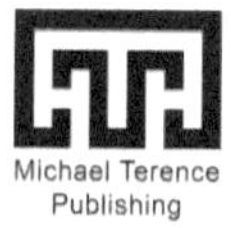

Contents

THE PREQUEL

The roots of my breakdown begin in my childhood. I had a pushy, manipulative mother and a bully of a father. And a brother seven years older than me. He had a different father. Something they didn't tell me until I was 21 years old. My mother always wanted me to emulate the achievements of my brother: pass the 11 plus, do Maths, Physics and Chemistry A levels, go to university, and become a Civil Engineer, just as he had done. She pursued this ambition with vigour.

At Junior School I could run like the wind and I loved football. I went on to be the fastest in Rugby and the third fastest in Warwickshire. In the Warwickshire Games I was placed third in the 100 yards. We crossed the line in a line all three of us with only 100th of a second between us. My time was 12 seconds. If my mother had left me alone, I would have gone on to be a professional footballer and a football manager.

My mother was not interested in my natural talents. Her first goal was for me to pass the 11 plus exam and go to Dunsmore Grammar School as my brother had done. To this effect, she managed to get me some extra homework to do when I was 10 years old. The headmaster hadn't wanted to give me the homework, but my mother went over his head and petitioned his boss.

The headmaster had selected 6 pupils who he thought would pass the 11 plus and was giving them extra lessons. My mother exposed this policy to Mr Donn, the headmaster's boss, and demanded that I was included in the six. Singling out only six pupils was against educational policy. If the press had found out, there would be hell. Mr Donn ordered the headmaster to give me extra lessons, but it made no difference. I failed the 11 plus anyway.

Most people would have given up at that, but not my mother. She set about finding a school in Rugby that did the 13 plus; a Secondary Modern School. Through sheer force of will and tenacity, she found one: a brand new school with an ambitious headmaster. But again, it made no difference. I failed the 13 plus anyway.

Most people would have given up at that, but not my mother. She wanted me to do O levels. The examination for secondary school pupils in the 1960s was CSEs - Certificates of Secondary Education. O Levels were reserved for grammar school pupils. Again, through her sheer force of will and tenacity, my mother persuaded the headmaster to enter me for O Levels, which he did, along with other boys in my class.

I passed 10 O levels at Grade 6. English with grade 4. I could now go to grammar school. I wanted to do A level English. It was my best subject but my mother and father overruled me. They said I must do Maths, Physics and Chemistry A levels as my brother had done. This time I fought back, at which my father put up his fists and said: 'Go on then, try it!' He used to do a bit of boxing when he was younger. He had hit me before when I objected to their plans. So I retreated to my bedroom and kept out of the way.

I was bottom of the class at grammar school and it soon became obvious to me that I was not going to get decent grades at A level. I tried to persuade my parents to let me go to Rugby Tech instead. I had taken O level Chemistry there. I liked their teaching methods and they treated you as a student, not a schoolboy. But my parents would not hear of it. My mother had worked hard to get me into grammar school, and she wasn't going to give that up. And my father's response was that if I were to go to Rugby Tech, I needn't think that I would live under his roof. What could I do? I didn't want to be homeless. I struggled on.

As I expected, I didn't get good grades at A level. I failed Physics and Chemistry and got grade E in Maths. My parents went mad. My father said I would have to retake them, to which I responded, there was no chance. So my father told me to get myself down to the Labour Exchange and sign on as a bricklayer. He said that that was all I was fit for. I retreated to my bedroom, crying.

There were a load of university prospectuses on my table. I swept them onto the floor, but one slim volume remained on the table. It was a prospectus for Trent Polytechnic. They would accept my one A level in Maths to enrol on an HND course in Building. I rang them up and enrolled the following week.

Thinking back, it was not a very good course; little of what I learned at Polytechnic was used in my working life. It was education for education's sake. I learned on the job.

It was a sandwich course, meaning I spent six months at college and six months in industry. My first job was Site Engineering. The problem was, I hadn't been told how to do it. I could use a dumpy level and a Theodolite, but I didn't know how to set out a building, how to put up profiles. The lecturer at Polytechnic used to work for Ordnance Survey, making maps. He taught us how to make maps, but he didn't teach us how to set out a building as he had never done it himself. I struggled on, but eventually after I graduated, my lack of knowledge got me the sack.

I was in charge of a site in Middlesbrough and I couldn't set out the position of drainage outlets in the concrete slab. So I kept putting back the pouring of the slab, trying to figure out how to position the drainage. I went home one Friday night. And on Monday morning when I got to site, the slab had been poured and I had got the sack. A foreman from another site had set the drainage outlets out on Saturday and they poured the slab that afternoon.

I had no choice but to go back home. My father told me that I needn't think he would be keeping me; that I had better get myself a job, that Automotive Products in Leamington Spa always wanted people, so I should get myself over there. I did. I got the job. It lasted 3 weeks. It was brutal. The noise was incredible, like 1000 cymbals being crashed together all day. I operated a machine that had four drills on it. I placed a wheel hub under the drill, pulled the handle and drilled four holes. That was it. That was the job. I did that all day and it numbed my brain.

I saw an advert in Building magazine. Shepherd Construction, in York, were looking for Trainee Estimators. I didn't mind Estimating at college, so I thought I would apply. At least I would be on a proper training course. I got the job. It was alright at first. I worked with an Estimator who taught me how to price drainage.

After a couple of years of training, I priced my first job. It was then that the pressure started. I was pricing a Bill of Quantities. Bills of Quantities are big. Some of them are over a foot thick. This one was 2 inches thick. You have to price every single rate in the Bill, and you only have two weeks to do it. Experienced Estimators could price quickly, but I was having to carefully workout my buildups for every rate, which made me slow. I worked extremely hard on that Bill of Quantities, but I didn't win the job. I came third. The group leader was pleased. He said it was a good market price and that I shouldn't want to win my first job. The average was that you would win one in 10.

I met Diane at the Bay Horse pub in Gillygate. They had a folk club there. I used to do a turn, sing a couple of songs. Diane used to work at the Electricity Board in Dundas Street. She was on the consumer unit answering questions from the public. She had a very nice telephone voice. Much later on, I rang her at work one day. I can't remember what it was about. Anyway, she spoke in a beautiful voice. She didn't normally use this voice when she spoke to me so I used to ring just to hear this voice. She soon cottoned on that it was me ringing though, and told me off for ringing her at work. Except one time she did that, it wasn't me, and she had told off a customer!

Maureen, who worked with Diane, had persuaded her to come to the folk club. Maureen and her husband also did a turn at the Bay Horse Folk Club. Diane was sat in the audience when I got up to do my turn. I sang Wild Flying Dove by Tom Paxton and Streets of London by Ralph McTell. They were two of my best songs. Diane asked Maureen who I was. Maureen didn't know, but she said she would find out. She spoke to the MC, who then told me of Diane's interest.

When Maureen and her husband got up to do their turn, I went and sat next to Diane. We fell into conversation very easily. She told me she worked at the Electricity Board and I told her I worked at Shepherd Construction. I described some of the work I did and she described her work. We talked about our interest in music. I said I liked The Beatles and she told me she had actually been to see them, twice. I was very jealous. I wanted to know all about it. She said it was pandemonium, lots of screaming girls and you could hardly hear The Beatles. I told her I'd seen lots of bands at Trent Polytechnic, but the best performer was a stand-up comic called Jasper Carrot. I told her some of his jokes, which is amazing for me because I usually can't tell jokes and I have a poor memory. But Diane just brought me out of myself.

I was usually quite shy with girls. But by the end of the night, I knew I had to see her again. And I didn't want to wait a week till the next folk club. So I asked her out for a meal at the Bernie Inn in the Windmill pub and she accepted.

We both had steak and chips, followed by ice cream and one of the famous Bernie Inn coffees: a frothy head over a black base. We talked and talked. Diane told me that she was separated from her husband, that he had made another woman pregnant and left her. She even told me how old she was, five years older than me. I told her some of my own history, including how I had signed a contract with a building company that allowed them to send me anywhere they wanted. And they did. So I was never long enough in one place to make friends. Consequently, I went out to pubs on my own and probably drank too much.

We left the Bernie Inn around 11:00 that night and I took Diane home in my yellow Triumph Herald. I loved that car. It went very well. That night I lost my virginity. Afterwards, we talked and talked and talked. And I floated back to my digs in Heworth at 4:00 in the morning.

I didn't see her again until the folk club on Thursday. Typical bloke: I expected more of what had happened the last time, but Diane wasn't playing ball. We did kiss though. Man, did we kiss. My lips were numb. I had kissed a girl before but nothing like this. It was degree level kissing. Again, we talked and talked and talked some more, and I floated back to my digs at 4:00 in the morning.

One of Diane's colleagues at work was going away for the weekend and needed someone to look after her Siamese cat while she was away. Diane volunteered and took me with her. But it didn't work out. We didn't like the cat, or should I say the cat didn't like us. Diane was in a funny mood and when I tried to kiss her, she slapped me across the face. I left her in the bedroom and retreated to the lounge. On our first full night together, we slept in separate beds.

That was typical of Diane. She was up and down. I put it down to the breakup of her marriage. She was taking Valium. She often hit me in those early days. We used to call it the BBC: the Battered Boyfriend Club. But I stuck with it and things did improve. If I'm honest, back then, I stuck with it because I had tasted the 'forbidden fruit' and I wasn't about to give it up.

We saw each other most nights. We used to go to a pub and sit talking all night with half a pint of lager, which was quite a change for me. Before I met Diane, I would have 5 or 6 pints regularly. I realise now I drank because I was lonely. But now I had Diane, I wasn't lonely, so I didn't need to drink so much.

The highlights were the holidays. We had some fantastic trips, Paris, Rome, Corfu, Dubrovnik, Majorca. Before the Paris trip, we stayed overnight in London. And Diane gave me a night I will never forget. She blew my mind, kept me awake all night. Majorca was my favourite trip. The hotel had been double booked, so someone else had our room. So we stayed the first night in another hotel, and checked into our proper room the next night. As compensation, the hotel gave us a cheap bottle of champagne. And both of us passed out. The champagne was so powerful we laid back, fully clothed, and slept. All I remember is waking up the next morning with a blinding headache, laid sideways on top of the bed with Diane next to me.

We went out together for five years before we were married. We had been driving in the car one day, not going very far, down Bishopthorpe Road, when I said to Diane: 'Are you going to marry me then?' She said: 'Well, you'll just have to wait and see!' Then she laughed and said: 'Alright', and I nearly knocked a man off his bike!

The more Bills I priced, the more the pressure increased. The Bills of Quantities were getting bigger. My biggest Bill was for a £6 million project called the Byker Wall in Newcastle, a council housing project. The pressure caused a pain in my stomach. I went to see the doctor. He said I had a nervous stomach that he could give me some tablets for it, but it wasn't a long term solution. That if I wasn't careful, I could develop an ulcer. I didn't tell Diane I was struggling at work at this point.

There was a recession on; Estimating was working flat out, pricing jobs, trying to get work. The area offices were laying people off. A Planning Surveyor came to work in Estimating from Darlington Area Office. The area manager at Darlington didn't have any work for him, but he was a good lad. Could we make use of him in Estimating? The Chief Estimator readily agreed to hire him on a temporary basis. Bruce, his name was. We had lunch together in the canteen. Bruce told me all about his job as a Planning Surveyor, and I liked the sound of it. Bruce loaned me some of his notes and I did some research on programming in the library.

The market picked up and I won my first job, an extension to a girls school in Leeds. I saw a job I fancied. Every month, a sheet was circulated in Estimating advertising vacancies for jobs. Gloucester area were advertising for a Planning Surveyor. I talked it over with my girlfriend, Diane. She had realised I struggled with the pressure and didn't like it in Estimating; she was supportive and wanted to help. So when I told her about the job in Gloucester as a Planning Surveyor, she encouraged me to go for it.

Funnily enough, despite the holidays where we shared a room, we never lived together. When I got the job, the move to Gloucester crystallised things.

We would get married and buy a house together there. It would be a new start, in another part of the country. We were very excited about it. Diane very much wanted to start a family.

But then there was hell on in Estimating.

They said they hadn't trained me for four years, only for me to up sticks and leave when I felt like it, which was fair enough. So I went to see the Chief Estimator. I have a bit of a silver tongue when I care to use it. We had a really good chat and I was totally honest with him. I told him I struggled with the pressure and I wanted to be involved in the building. I wanted to build something rather than just to price it. We en ded the interview with the Chief Estimator shaking my hand and saying that he had no doubt I could do the job as a Planning Surveyor and wished me well in my new career. And so I moved to Gloucester 6 months before our wedding.

We were married at York Registry Office on 28th of September 1979. My parents did not approve of my choice of wife. They did not like the fact that Diane had been married before, which is ironic considering my mother had been married before she met my father. My brother Chris never made it to our wedding. I can't remember what his excuse was. Basically, he couldn't be bothered. That was always his attitude to me. He always had something more important to do. My sister Julie came though.

It was a lovely day. The sun shone. It was a nice service and a nice building, the Registry Office, and they had a garden at the back. I remember the roses were full of flowers. Photographs were taken and we went off to a reception at a hotel.

We didn't have a honeymoon. Our honeymoon was moving into our new home. A semi-detached bungalow in Newent. It was a beautiful site situated in the grounds of what used to be a stately home with big mature trees. The soil was fantastic, you could grow anything. I remember I bought some cauliflower plug plants from a garden centre, planted them at the side of the bungalow and they grew into massive cauliflowers. People used to stop and stare at them.

We started practising for a baby straight away. Diane didn't look for a job. She said there wasn't any point; that she would be looking after the baby. On reflection now, I think it would have been better if she had found a job. I would come home and she would be sat on the floor in the lounge. She did do some decorating though.

The job was great. I really enjoyed Planning. I had a good Site Manager called Ivor. I was working on a Shepherd development site: Advanced Factories in Coleshill.

Diane was still very keen to start a family. But after six months of trying, she still wasn't pregnant. I was tested and was alright, which meant the problem must be Diane.

I was very happy at Gloucester area office and I didn't want to leave but, unfortunately they had a big job at the SAS headquarters that was losing money. The job I was working on was making money, but it wasn't enough to offset the losses on the SAS contract. So a decision was made by the Managing Director, Anthony Herd, to close the office. The Gloucester area manager, Mr House, personally arranged for my transfer to York. He did not want Shepherds to lose me. York area office paid for my removal expenses, all arranged by Mr House. So I was moved to York area office.

What I hadn't realised was that York Area office didn't really want me. They gave me a tough time at first. My wages were kept deliberately low, pay rises were minimal. I very nearly packed it in and went back to Gloucester. I would have had to find another job, but that was preferable to how I was being treated in York.

We were initially staying in Diane's mother and father's house, while we sold the semi- detached bungalow in Newent, for a healthy profit, enabling us to buy a detached bungalow in York, for only a small increase in the mortgage. The doctor in York referred Diane to the hospital, to have her fallopian tubes 'blown out' We were still staying with Diane's parents when Diane had the procedure, which was fortunate as it meant that her parents could look after her when she was recovering from the operation. But, while she was on the operating table, the consultant found she had endometriosis, a growth in the womb. They decided to operate immediately, and gave Diane another dose of anaesthetic and performed the operation, cutting her stomach open to gain access to the womb.

Myself, Diane and her parents were all shocked by the operation. We never imagined anything like that would happen. I was at work at the time, thinking she was just in for a minor operation, when I got to the hospital and found her in intensive care, I got the shock of my life. They nearly lost her. I nearly lost her. They couldn't get her temperature back up. They wrapped her in a metallic blanket. Eventually her temperature did rise, but it was touch and go for a while.

I was shocked when I went in to see her in hospital, but not as shocked as she was. All the colour had gone from her face. She was unconscious. My foot touched something by her bed. It was a plastic bag full of blood. The consultant came to see us. She said she had removed as much of the endometriosis as she could, so that now was the best time to try for a baby, before it came back. It was not a case of 'if' but 'when' the endometriosis came back. Diane's wound was sealed with metal clips and so I asked the nurse about trying for a baby now; I was very worried about disturbing them if we had sex. But the nurse reassured me they would not come out.

When Diane came home from hospital, we did try for a baby again, but we were not successful. Over 10 years, Diane had her stomach cut open three more times to remove the endometriosis. On the third time, it became a full hysterectomy. They even removed her appendix. So that was the end of trying for a baby. We were devastated at not being able to have children, but we were both just glad Diane was still alive.

We had been through so much with the three operations. We just needed a little peace and quiet to gather ourselves after such trauma. We were disappointed we could not have a child, but we tackled Diane's health problems together and it brought us closer. When we were ready, we would try for adoption.

On the plus side, I enjoyed my job as a Planning Surveyor and to my surprise, I was good at it. I used my Estimating experience to calculate the length of operations on the Contract Programme. My Contract Programmes were very accurate. Some of the younger Site Managers appreciated them, but there was an attitude amongst the older Site Managers that the programme was something you hung on the wall and ignored.

The doctor put Diane on HRT tablets and for a while she enjoyed a period of good health. She put on weight. Although she wasn't strong enough to get a job, I used to come home to a proper home cooked meal every night, so I started putting on weight too! We applied to adopt a child but by this stage we were told we were too old: Diane was 45 and I was 40. We didn't push it. I was just glad to have Diane back to some health and happiness. Things carried on like that for a while, until Diane developed neck pain.

The doctor said she had a trapped nerve in her neck. He booked her on a course of traction in the hospital. Basically, they sat her in a chair, fitted a collar around her neck and stretched her neck upwards, to try and release the nerve. It didn't work. In fact, it made it worse. As well as neck pain, Diane had pain in her extremities, in her hands and feet. The fingers of her left hand curled over and pressed into the palm of her hand. The doctor said she had neuropathy. They could cut the tendons in her hand to release her fingers, but she wouldn't be able to use the hand again. It would just flop about. At that time, she still had use of her thumb and forefinger, so she decided against the operation.

My luck had run out at work too. Previously all my jobs had made money but I was put on a job that was losing money, a £6 million building society in Harrogate. It was losing half a million pounds. They were looking for a scapegoat and they picked on me. I was made redundant. Diane burst into tears, but I was too angry for tears.

I got another job fairly quickly as an Estimator for a small building company. I had kept my Estimating notes and slipped back into it quite easily. But I couldn't come to terms with being made redundant. I couldn't accept that I would never plan another job. I lasted 6 months and had my first breakdown.

It took me a year to recover, during which Diane was very supportive and fought hard for me to have the best care. As luck would have it, a lad that I used to work with was working for a firm in Ilkley and they needed a Planner. It should have been the dream job. All they wanted me to do was draw up Construction Programmes, which I loved doing. But I wasn't fully recovered from the breakdown. I lasted a year before I had another breakdown. Diane rang Bootham Park Hospital and asked to speak to Dr Pal, the psychiatrist who had treated me before. He agreed to admit me straight away and Diane's father took me there in his car.

It took two years to recover from that one. My psychiatrist told me in no uncertain terms that I must not go back into Planning. It was too stressful.

He suggested I got a job in a shop, which I did. I worked for Oxfam as a volunteer for six months. Then I got a job selling suitcases for six months. Then a job in menswear at Browns and finally a job selling garden furniture at the McArthur Glen shopping centre.

During this time, Diane's health was getting worse. She was spending increased amounts of time lying in bed. It was the only way she could stop the pain. Any movement set the pain off. We reached a point where she was crying with pain when I went to work and still crying with pain when I came home. The neuropathy got worse. Both her feet twisted and she could not stand. It reached a point where she became totally bedbound. She would pass the time reading, so we bought her a Kindle.

I couldn't bear the thought of her going to a home, so I gave up work to look after her. We applied for Disability Living Allowance and Diane received the maximum amount, yet we still had to dip into our savings. We had carers at first but they rushed in and rushed out, leaving me to clear up their mess. So it became easier for me to look after her myself, which is what I did; for 15 years.

With Diane now bedbound, it was left to me to look after the house. She showed me a few recipes and I went on a cookery course: 'Cooking for Men', and bought a Mary Berry Recipe book. I enjoyed cooking and began to treat it as a hobby. It was the same with cleaning and ironing – I enjoyed it. I did everything on my own with no outside help from family or friends.

We learned that Diane had bowel cancer. She did a test and it was confirmed. But she was so ill, she couldn't stand the thought of going into hospital for any treatment. It was too much on top of her existing conditions. She eventually died of bowel cancer.

We were together for 45 years. I couldn't handle her dying. Caring for her had been my whole world for the last 15 years. Her death tipped me into a third breakdown. I will tell the story of that starting in the next chapter.

THE THIRD

BREAKDOWN

One

I was imprisoned in a secure mental hospital. What was my crime? My wife died and I had a breakdown. This was my third breakdown. For the first two, I was a voluntary patient, allowed to come and go as I pleased. They treated me humanely. This time they Sectioned me, which gave them the power to keep me locked up for six months. Which is what they did.

The day after Diane died, I knew I was having a breakdown. I recognised the signs. My mind was racing out of control. I moved too quickly. I spoke too quickly. I said crazy things. I went to see my neighbour and said: 'I'm giving you my car, I don't need it anymore. I'm buying an electric car '. I gave my neighbours my wife Diane's bottle of Chanel #5 perfume. I had a test drive in a VW ID 3 electric car. I rang up an electrician to give me a quotation for an electric car charging point. I rang up a house clearance company and cleared out everything in my garage, including a ladder which I needed to clean the fascia on my house. Those are just a sample of what I did in the immediate aftermath of Diane's death. My mind was buzzing night and day. I pestered the life out of my neighbour. When I came out of hospital he didn't want anything to do with me. I had treated him so badly during my breakdown. I apologised. I told him I couldn't help it. But he is not the friend he used to be anymore.

If Diane had still been alive, she would have recognised the signs and rung the doctor. But I didn't have anybody. I was completely alone. I walked down to the doctor's surgery. It was shut. So I walked to the surgery in Acomb, about 6 miles. I didn't go in the car because I didn't trust myself to drive. I was too bad. I didn't have an appointment. I said to the receptionist that my wife had died and I was having a breakdown. Could I see a doctor? I need to be admitted to Moss Park Hospital. She told me to sit and wait. Eventually, a doctor did come. This was at the height of the COVID epidemic. The Doctor was all masked up with PPE. I can't remember exactly what he said, but the upshot of it was he refused to send me to Moss Park. I found myself out on the street. It was cold, very cold.

I staggered down the street and collapsed in front of the supermarket. The next thing I remember is sitting on a bench inside Morrisons supermarket and someone giving me a cup of tea. A taxi came and took me home. I've no idea who paid for it. I had no money on me.

So I was back to square one at home. I asked my neighbour to take me to Moss Park but he refused. There is a chap at the end of the cul-de-sac who is always friendly, so I knocked on his door and asked him to ring for a taxi to take me to Moss Park. They were getting ready to see their granddaughter, but they did ring. The taxi did come. But once again, I have no idea who paid for it.

When we got to the hospital, it was shut. I banged on the door, but they took no notice, so I lay down on the cold pavement outside the big glass doors. This was too much for the taxi driver. He got out of his cab and banged on the door. This time they did answer the door. I remember the taxi driver shouting at them saying they must admit me, which they did reluctantly.

I have no memory of what happened after that. The next thing I remember is I'm in another hospital in Scarborough and they're preparing to Section me. I tried to prove that I was sane by describing the most difficult job I have done: the reroofing of Terry's Chocolate Factory. But they weren't listening. Their eyes had glazed over. They Sectioned me.

Normally I'm a friendly, funny kind of guy, but when I'm having a breakdown, I am the opposite. I shout and scream and say all sorts of crazy things. I call this person 'the other person' because it is not me talking. It is the illness talking. Yes, I was a handful, but it did not justify the way they treated me.

During the first two breakdowns, as a voluntary patient, I could come and go as I wished. I was in hospital for 10 weeks in both cases. For the last two weeks I was allowed to go home for the weekend. This time though, my third breakdown, I was not allowed to go anywhere. All the doors and windows were locked shut. When I ventured out of my bedroom, I was told to 'go and lay on your bed'. I spent a lot of time laying on my bed. It was a very uncomfortable bed, rock hard with a slippery plastic mattress cover. When I was allowed out of my bedroom, they kept a close eye on me. All it needed was a trigger to set me off screaming and shouting. Some of the healthcare assistants only had to look at me and it would trigger me. But I wasn't like that all the time. Sometimes I was quite calm. I'd say it was about 50:50. 50% calm, 50% 'the other person'.

When I was having an episode, they took it upon themselves to grab hold of me. I quickly learned that the best way to stop them hurting me was to play dead and fall on the floor. This gave rise to another tactic of theirs. I was sat quietly in the common area when four of the assistants jumped on me, dragged me onto the floor, ripped my jeans down and injected me in my bottom. This happened quite often.

Before the 3rd breakdown, I was taking Quetiapene. It was a good drug. It kept me calm and acted like a sleeping tablet. I always slept well on this medication. The hospital took me off this and put me on a cocktail of drugs which did not keep me calm and did not help me sleep. Consequently, I was awake most of the night. I had no entertainment, no books, no papers, nothing to do. Just lay on my back. It gave me a back ache. I suffered for backache for six months after I was released, but it's OK now.

My mind was in turmoil. My nerves were jangling. I couldn't keep still. Goodness knows how I passed the time. Mercifully, I have very little memory of that time. I do remember going to an arts and crafts room and colouring in pictures, drawing pictures and making things with a couple of games.

Most of the time I was dressed in pyjamas. My clothes had gone missing, along with all my possessions, my wallet, phone, bank cards, wedding ring, watch. Even the laces in my shoes had been removed.

I was diagnosed as bipolar. I do go very high, but I don't go low. I have not had depression, thank goodness. The diagnosis of my first breakdown was hypomania. Which is a mild form of mania. There is nothing minor about my mania. After my second breakdown, I researched my illness on the computer. The best match I could make was schizophrenia, but that didn't explain everything. Then I came across a form of schizophrenia called 'split personality' - it's very rare - in which the patient behaves independently as two different people, and that is what I did.

I was like a hot potato that the hospitals passed to one another. Moss Park passed me on to Scarborough. Scarborough passed me on to Doncaster. Doncaster passed me on to Darlington. Darlington passed me on to Newcastle Royal Infirmary. Newcastle passed me back to Darlington. Darlington passed me back to Moss Park in York. I have very little memory of these hospitals. The only one I can really remember is my second visit to Moss Park.

I do remember being in Newcastle Royal Infirmary on a hospital trolley, being held down by two guards. Apparently, I had an operation on my stomach in that hospital but I can't remember much about it. I remember being in a hospital bed guarded by a big black nurse who wouldn't let me out of bed to go to the toilet. Consequently, I wet myself. He cleaned me up with lots of wipes. Very roughly. I was a prisoner.

I was transferred to Moss Park for a second time on Christmas Eve 2022. I had COVID and was kept in isolation, laid on my bed for a month. They kept testing me, putting a swab up my nose. Fortunately, they did give me a radio tuned to Greatest Hits Radio. It was great and I really enjoyed listening to that.

When I was in Doncaster Mental Hospital, I was told that I could apply to challenge my Section to have it removed. They filled in the form, I signed it and off it went. I was told at Moss Park that the Tribunal would be held on 8th of February 23. I was allowed an advocate and a solicitor. I met with both of them. They both said I stood a good chance of overturning this Section, but we didn't discuss tactics. It was just a 'get to know you' meeting.

There was one of the guards who particularly disliked me. I'll call him 'the nasty white man'. His favourite move was the arm lock. The first time he did it to me, he really hurt me. I thought he was going to break my arm. He gripped really tight. The second time I was ready for him. I fell to the ground before he could get a good grip.

The funniest time was in the office. They didn't like patients coming into the office. I can't remember why I was there, but I do remember Nasty White Man shouting, 'get out of the office'. He went for me, grabbed my arm and I went down like a sack of potatoes. So now they had a problem. I was laid right in the middle of the office and they had to step over me to get to their seats. And I was going nowhere. I wanted to see how they would get out of this one. After much discussion, they fetched a blue sheet that they rolled me on to. Then they inflated it with a foot pump. Then all four of them dragged me out of the door. It was hilarious. Of course, as soon as I was out of the office, I stood up.

In January, they gave me some of my possessions back: my wallet, cards and money, my watch and my phone. My phone was flat and I didn't have a charger. It was a pay- as-you-go phone. I usually topped it up with my card at the Post Office. There was a Post Office in New Earswick. I asked if I could go there and top up my phone. To my amazement, they agreed. I should also mention they gave me back my wedding ring.

So now I could make phone calls. The first thing I did was ring the doctors, but as soon as they found out I was in Moss Park, they wouldn't make an appointment. So I thought, right, I'll make a private appointment. The Nuffield Hospital is right next to Moss Park. I rang them up and made an appointment to see a doctor next week. So now all I had to do was to get leave from Moss Park. I made-up a story about going to see a podiatrist about a veruca on my foot. I said I had been waiting a year and I didn't want to miss it and they fell for it hook, line and sinker.

They said: Yes, of course I could see my podiatrist, but as I am banned from using the taxi firm, I would have to go on the bus, which was fine by me. Why was I banned by the taxi firm? I reported a taxi driver for swearing at me using the F word. It backfired on me. I said the F word on the phone, in quoting exactly what the taxi driver said, but it somehow got transposed and they thought I was swearing at them, so they banned me. Which was a bit awkward as the hospital only use this taxi firm. They didn't have a contract with anyone else.

I went to see the doctor and said I would like the drugs in my prescription that I was taking before my breakdown. The doctor made an excuse and left the surgery. When she came back she had rung Moss Park and they were sending a car for me.

But I didn't give up. I made an appointment to see another private doctor. Things were improving. I had been out on leave with a guard into town to buy some clothes. Most of my clothes had been stolen. I bought 2 pairs of trousers, some shirts and boxer shorts from Marks and Spencer. I had a couple more successful leaves and they were pleased with me.

So I asked if I could have leave to go home. There were lots of things I had to do. To my amazement, they agreed. I said I would organise the taxi. I used a different firm but instead of going home I went to see the doctor. I described my treatment at Moss Park, the wrong drugs, the attacks by Nasty White Man, keeping me locked up. She was very sympathetic. She examined me for bruises, but there weren't any. I don't bruise easily. But she was so concerned by the treatment, she said she would report the case to Safeguarding. I left feeling very pleased and caught a taxi back to Moss Park.

I was busy preparing my case for the Tribunal. I asked my solicitor and advocate to come and see me. But for some reason - I'm not sure what - they were reluctant to come. On another unescorted visit to town, I called in at the private doctors to see how they were getting on with the Safeguarding case. I can't remember the exact details of the meeting, but it became obvious to me that they had taken my money (£200) and done nothing. It triggered me. I started shouting at them. I stormed out of the office and fell down the steps, landing flat on my face in the cobbled yard.

My solicitor did not come and see me until half an hour before the Tribunal started. Obviously. I did not then have time to brief her. I told her exactly what I thought of her performance. With this ringing in her ears, she went in to the Tribunal. I did not go to the Tribunal for two reasons. One, I would have to do the solicitor's work for her, as she had not been briefed. And two, if the judge said something that triggered me, and I reacted, they would never let me out.

I lost the Tribunal. Dr David Brine, the consultant Psychiatrist reported to the tribunal that he had been contacted by a private doctor in Stonegate who said that I had spat at him. This was the doctor I had been to see. I did not spit at him. I've never spat at anyone. All I could think of was that I do make quite a lot of saliva. Perhaps that is what he saw. The tribunal turned on this so-called spitting incident. It was all the proof they needed to refuse to lift the Section.

Two

I was back to square one and it looked like I would have to serve the full six months of my Section, and there was no guarantee that it would not be extended for another six months. I needed to change tack. I decided on a charm offensive. I was a good boy. I didn't shout and scream. I didn't bang on the office door. I even offered to show them some yoga exercises I had devised. One of them did actually take up my offer.

I started going to church. I went with two guards initially, gradually reducing to one. Timing was a problem. I was only allowed one hour leave, but the church service lasts over an hour, so I was always late, which didn't go down well. But still we were making progress. One of these leaves had a bizarre ending.

We had been out on home leave. One of the healthcare assistants had brought me in the hospital's car and was picking me up in an hour's time. All went well until when we returned to the hospital and parked up. I didn't feel like going to my room immediately so I sat in the car whilst the others got out. And it sort of escalated. Somebody came and sat next to me trying to persuade me to get out of the car. They sent for reinforcements. I counted seven of them at one point. They opened the door and tried to drag me on to a wheelchair. I extended my legs and went as stiff as a board.

They wrestled me on to the cold, hard tarmac and four of them pinned me down. It was winter, February, and it was cold. Very cold. My shirt had risen up, exposing bare flesh. We stayed like this for quite a while. I can't remember what I said, but they did release their grip. I stood up, ran to the doors of the hospital, and straight to my room. Leave was cancelled for a couple of weeks after that.

I was punched in the face by one of the inmates. This inmate was arguing with one of the nurses. I got up from the table and stood in front of him, protecting the nurse. He punched me in the face, sent me flying over a chair. My head hit the floor hard. I was knocked out, only for a short while, but when I came round I was seeing stars. I knew that was concussion from when I played rugby. I was examined by a doctor, but they didn't do anything. They never do. So I rang 999 and reported the assault, but as soon as they found out I was in a mental hospital, they put the phone down.

I had been punched in the face before at Doncaster. The same thing happened there. The police put the phone down. Altogether, the police put the phone down on me five times on 999 calls. I rang 111 fourteen times, with the same result. When you are Sectioned in a mental hospital, they can do anything they want to you and you are powerless to stop them. They can almost literally get away with murder.

I have a brother, Chris, in London. He is my next of kin. He rang the hospital from time to time to see how I was getting on, but he didn't speak to me. It was him that organised my wife Diane's funeral, although I had no idea this was happening. Nobody told me, not even Chris; he just did it – and even paid for it. I was devastated to learn that the staff at the hospital were refusing me permission not only to organise the funeral but I was even refused permission to attend my own wife's funeral.

I saw part of the funeral on a laptop computer from Doncaster Mental Hospital. It was a travesty of the funeral I had planned for Diane. Only four people attended, all neighbours, no family went, not even my brother who had organised it. I also have a sister, Julie, who lives in London, and my mother, who is 96, who lives in a care home in Rugby. Neither of them came to the funeral.

Chris had Diane cremated. And I was so outraged at this that I decided to write a proper memorial service for her and give her the sendoff she deserved. And this is what I've done. I wrote three new songs, added two old songs and recorded them all with the Royal Philharmonic Orchestra. Let me tell you the story.

I have written so many songs, 130 in total, in so many different styles. It would take half a dozen bands to do them all. So I thought, what I needed was an orchestra. Orchestras can play any type of music. So I searched the internet for orchestras and the Royal Philharmonic Orchestra came up. So I gave them a call. A very nice lady answered the phone. I started to explain that I was organising a memorial service for Diane and I needed an orchestra to play the music. But I didn't get very far until the tears came, she said. Not to worry that they would do everything they could to help me and that she would get the manager of the orchestra to ring me and he would tell me what he needed.

And so he did. His name is Ian Clay. He said he needed a proper studio recorded demo and it would cost £20,000 for the five songs. And so I googled recording studios and Baker Land Studios in Leeds came up. Andy Bake said yes, he could do a studio recorded demo. So this is what I have done.

I was discharged from hospitalon the 11th of April 2023. The first recording session in Baker Land Studios was on the 2nd of May. I went to see Ian Clay at Abbey Road Studios on 13th of May. He showed me around and explained how they made a recording. I recorded the five tracks with the Royal Philharmonic Orchestra on 3rd of July 2023. The second 6 tracks we recorded on 7th of September.

Diane's memorial service was held on 28th September 2023, our 44th wedding anniversary, at Saint James the Deacon Church in Woodthorpe. I decided, after all this effort, that I wanted a proper grave and a headstone for Diane. So I had her ashes disinterred, bought a plot in Fulford Cemetery, and had a headstone made. I now have somewhere I can go to remember her. I would not have done that if I had been allowed to go to Diane's funeral.

My biological family are not close. I have my brother Chris, who lives in London, and sister Julie, who also lives in London. On my release from hospital, I made a point of trying to talk to my brother as often as possible on the phone. He rarely rings me. I also said I wanted to see him. I did the same with Julie, but she refuses to see me. I'm conscious of the fact that since Diane died, I'm on my own, her mother and father died some years ago.

They were my family, so I've tried to rekindle connections with my biological family.

I have begun rehearsals for a second album in London with a pianist called Clive Dunn, which means visits to London every fortnight. I've used these visits to London to see Chris. He frequently has other things to do, but we have managed three visits so far, so the signs are promising. But Julie remains elusive. My mother in the care home has dementia. I don't think she knew who I was the last time I visited her.

Three

My grandfather came from Switzerland. He was the oldest of four brothers. My father tells the story that he sold his inheritance for a shilling and came to England. My father always thought that he had been cheated out of his inheritance, which set me thinking. Those brothers must have had families. They were relatives of mine. They were family. Could I make contact with them and form a Swiss branch of the family?

I told them at the hospital that I wanted to visit my Swiss family as soon as I could. I made no secret of the fact that that was my ambition. And I started planning. I was doing so well that my leave was extended from one hour to two hours to three hours to six hours. As I was planning my trip, I was very careful not to exceed these times. Indeed, for the six hour one, I came back an hour early. These were all unescorted leaves.

First of all I needed a passport. I went to the Post Office in Smiths in Coney St and obtained a passport form. I filled it in, had my photograph taken at Tesco and took the completed form back to Smiths. I gave the assistant the story that I wanted to visit my Swiss grandfather, that he had terminal cancer and they didn't know how long he had left. The assistant said she would fast track it for me. Everyone said it would take 10 weeks to get a passport. I got mine in 10 days.

On one of my leaves, at home, I packed a suitcase. I was ready. All I needed was another unescorted leave. It was unfortunate that the last unescorted leave I had had, I came back a quarter of an hour late and they didn't like that. I apologised profusely, said I didn't realise the time, which was true. But all leave was cancelled for a while. The problem was they didn't have enough staff to give me escorted leave and, of course, I had broken the rules by being late back from unescorted leave.

One day they decided I could have two hour's unescorted leave the following day at 9:00. But on the morning, my leave was cut to one hour unescorted. I walked to the bus stop at 9:30 and boarded a bus for the train station. At 10:00 I hired a taxi to take me home to collect my suitcase and then take me back to the railway station. At 11:00 I boarded a train for Manchester. At 12:30 I boarded a bus to Manchester Airport.

I did not have a ticket to Zurich. I selected a guard at the airport and spun him the tale about my Swiss grandfather dying of cancer. I said I wasn't very good on a computer. Was it possible to buy a ticket at the airport? He was superb. He took me to the Swiss Air Terminal, waited until I had bought my ticket and took me to the queue for the airline. I caught the 3:00 flight to Zurich. We landed at 4:30. There was an hour time difference.

At 4:30. I asked a taxi driver to take me to the nearest hotel and I arrived at the Novotel, near to the airport at 5:00 PM. At 6:00 PM I went shopping at a mini supermarket in Zurich and bought sandwiches, buns, milk and a cold cappuccino. At 6:30, I ate the sandwich on a pavement bench in Zurich. At 8:00 I climbed into bed, but I could not sleep. I had no drugs with me. This was Saturday 18th of March 2023: D-Day.

Sunday 19th March 2023: D-day plus one. 6:00 AM Breakfast at Novotel Zurich.

6:40 AM Train to Zurich airport.

7:30 Train to Solothurn, where my Swiss family come from. 9:00 Arrive at Solothurn.

10:30 Bus to Kirche ze Kreuzen Church.

In the hotel, I had asked the receptionist to Google churches in Solothurn and he came up with the above church.

10:45 Arrive at Kirche ze Kreuzen Church.

10:48 Burst into tears when the people were kind to me.

They took me into their church and sat me next to a man who could speak a little English. The service was in German, which I didn't understand of course, but the priest who played the piano was like a concert pianist. He was brilliant. I really enjoyed that service and even took communion.

12 noon Finish service, taken into church hall and given orange juice, bread and cheese.

I explained that I was looking for my Swiss family who came from Solothurn. I wondered if there was any record of them in the parish register. They said they would have a look. The Parish Register turned out to be a big book, three inches thick, dating back hundreds of years. I left them looking through the book and went to catch a bus back to Solothurn at 2:00 PM.

2:30 PM I caught a train back to Zurich.

3:30 PM I arrive in Zurich.

The train I had caught took me into the centre of Zurich, whereas my hotel was near the airport at the outskirts of the city. I was hungry but spotted a Burger King and had a hamburger and chips and a cappuccino. It was 4:00 PM. At 4:30 I caught a taxi to the Novotel, but he took me to the one in the city. It cost me 80 francs to get him to take me to the Novotel by the airport.

6:00 PM Arrived at the Novotel.

I was hungry again. I had spotted an Italian restaurant on my way to the supermarket last night. I went in and had a lasagna. It was superb. It cost 36 francs. It was 7:00 PM. 9:00 PM bed at Novotel, but again couldn't sleep.

Monday 20th March 2023 D-Day +2. No sleep at all last night.

6:00 AM breakfast at Novotel Zurich.

7:00 AM Walk to the Post Office to post letters to Doctor Brine and to the Church I had visited in Solothurn. I wrote to Doctor Brine, telling him where I was. I wrote to the Church asking them to post any information about my Swiss family to my home address in York. The receptionist told me that the Post Office opened at 7:00 AM but when I got there, I found a sign which said they open at 9:00 AM. I used the two hours to walk around the area and buy teabags, sandwiches and coke for dinner at Zurich airport.

9:00 AM Posted letters, walked back to Novotel. 9:30 AM Lay on bed, very tired but could not sleep. 10:00 Packed suitcase.

10:30 Had a cup of tea and checked out of the hotel. 11:00 Tram to Zurich Airport.

11:30 Brought a ticket to Manchester Airport. The flight takes off at 5:00 this evening. Used the time to have a haircut, buy a shirt, eat my sandwich and buns and milk and look around the 'Circle shops'.

2:30 PM In departure lounge waiting for flight to Manchester.

5:00 PM Flight delayed.

6:00 PM Boarded plane to Manchester Airport.

When I boarded, I noticed some very nice leather seats on the left hand side with no one sitting in them. So I sat down there. People were filing past me. The plane was filling up. A member of the cabin crew moved me to my proper seat. Apparently I was sat in first class. Without my medication for some days now, I was very high. I could talk for England! I had a brilliant conversation with my neighbour on the plane. She came from Manchester. I asked her if she knew any recording studios in Manchester. She did. Her husband was a musician. I explained that I wanted to make an album.

7:30 PM Flight landed at Manchester Airport. One of the cabin crew came up to me and asked me to accompany her. Two policemen, a man and a woman, were waiting for me. I asked them if they were going to put cuffs on me. They said that wouldn't be necessary. The male policeman didn't think I had any luggage. He started to walk away from baggage claim. I told him I had a suitcase and waited for it to come round the carousel. They took me to the police station where I asked if they were arresting me. The female police officer said that they weren't. They just needed to get me back to Moss Park Hospital and that a car was waiting if I would follow them.

As I said before, I was so high I could talk for England. We had a cracking conversation on that journey back to York. Everyone told their life stories. The female police officer was mad on vintage cars. The male police officer used to work on building sites, same as me. We talked and talked and talked for the full 2 hours it took to drive to York. I really enjoyed that drive. It was the highlight of the trip.

8:00 PM taken to police station.

8:15 PM Commence the drive to Moss Park Hospital 10:00 PM Arrived at Moss Park Hospital.

10:10 PM Given meds by Jasmine: Olanzapine 20mgs (antipsychotic drug); Zopiclone

3.75mgs (sleeping tablet) and Larazepan 1mg, (same family as Valium).

10:30 PM Went to sleep.

6:30 AM Woke after a good night's sleep, the first sleep since the day before D-Day. 7:00 AM Breakfast: Rice Krispies and a cup of tea. This was Zurich time. I had lost an hour. And it's now

8:10 AM. Waiting for main breakfast of porridge when the canteen opens at 9:00 AM.

Meanwhile, back at Moss Park, on the morning of my departure, everything was in turmoil. I didn't return at 10:30 AM as planned. This was nothing unusual; I had often been late coming back. By 11:30 they were getting worried. I had said I was going to the cafe in the Post Office at New Earswick. One of the healthcare assistants went to look for me there. When she drew a blank, someone was dispatched to my house. She knocked on the door and peered through the windows, but there was no sign of life.

Somebody - probably Doctor Brine - wondered if I had gone to Switzerland since I had made no secret of the fact that I wanted to go there, but they couldn't see how I could have managed it. It seemed impossible. Doctor Brine had said they'd give it an hour and then they'd have to ring the police.

I don't know for sure that this account is accurate. I've pieced it together from what I was told when I got back, but it was something like that.

They rang the police and told them that one of their patients was missing. I don't know the full story, but they found my name on a flight out to Zurich. But they were too late. I had already left. They contacted Interpol who found me on a flight out of Zurich bound for Manchester Airport. Two policemen were dispatched to intercept me on the plane, which was great. It saved me having to catch the train. I wanted to be back in Moss Park Hospital. I had not had any meds since I left, and my mind was speeding out of control.

Four

They treated me much better after that. I had proved beyond a reasonable doubt that I could manage perfectly well on my own. I had done something that they thought I could not do, that they thought was impossible. Five weeks later, I was released.

The law relating to being Sectioned needs to be changed. It is too powerful. It gives doctors carte blanche to do anything they want to you. In a civilised society this cannot be allowed to continue.

An independent doctor needs to be appointed to supervise the treatment of mental patients under Section, reviewed every week. Doctor Brine was too powerful. He ruled like a dictator. No one person should have so much power. Decisions should be made democratically, by all the nurses and doctors involved in the patient's treatment.

Only in exceptional cases should anyone be imprisoned under lock and key when they are no danger to society. I do not disagree with accompanied leave. I got on very well with my guards, but there is an important principle at stake here: Sectioned mental patients are not prisoners in jail. But that is how the present regime treats them.

Doctor Brine released me from my Section on Tuesday 11th of April 2023. I had been held under lock and key for 22 weeks. Since then I have managed perfectly well at home on my own, as I knew I would.

Everybody at Moss Park was talking about 'D-Day'. Someone there said that anyone who can escape from this lot should not be in here.

Does the end justify the means? Well, it has certainly been traumatic. I'm cured, as much as I will ever be: my mind is calm most of the time. My nerves have stopped jangling. My brain works alright. I have been able to plan Diane's memorial service and start my business: The STU COMPANY 725 Limited. I could not have done that if I had not recovered.

But there can be no excuse for the abusive treatment I suffered. The mental health professionals managed perfectly well during my first and second breakdowns without resorting to violence or locking me up. I feel if Diane had still been alive to advocate for me as she had done previously, none of this would have happened. They were only able to do it as I was on my own. Yes, I have a brother, but all he did was ring the ward and have a cosy chat with the nurse. He never spoke to me. The police did not want to know. Citizens Advice did not want to know. The solicitor didn't want to know, and the advocate didn't want to know.

Five

THE NOTEBOOKS - TRANSCRIPTION

I would like to talk to a senior manager or a ward sister.

According to this leaflet, 'Your rights under the Mental Health Act, Section 5: Detention of Patients already in Hospital.

I don't remember being Sectioned. I have never been Sectioned in my life. I came into hospital readily. I don't like hospitals. Nobody does. But I recognised that I was having a breakdown. And I had no alternative but to be brought into hospital. In this instance, I do not remember being admitted.

The reason for that is that I can operate as two independent people. I cannot remember the name for it, but Professor Weiss in Zurich says it is one in many millions. In 25 years of practise, I was the only case he had come across. He says he cannot cure me, but he can show me how to live with it. I should be in Geneva now, but I was persuaded that I would get better treatment here.

I have been in many hospitals all over the world during the past 20 years. This hospital is the worst I have ever been in. Normally I never complain, but I cannot leave this.

I was admitted at 10:00 last night. I have not had anything to eat in all that time and it is now 1:45. One of the nurses has finally made me a bowl of soup. I am speechless.

You have not seen the last of me. I've asked if I can be a cleaner. I love cleaning. I particularly love ironing. I don't want paying for the work. I have plenty of money. It is the occupancy. I need something to occupy my hands without taxing my brain.

I am not going to apply for a job as a cleaner. I'm not going to send this to a barrister, provided you learn the lessons. If you don't, I will send it to a barrister.

I'm actually very grateful for all the aggro. It has cured me. Well, not cured, but it is a start and I want to pay you back for it. I do have money, but I don't want to give you money. I want to give you my time.

I think a doctor did turn up this morning. He looked very prosperous. Smart suit, nails cut. He said he could see me for 5 minutes. I burst out laughing. I hate people like that. They're ripping off the NHS.

Best tomato soup I've ever had.

This doctor refuses to write down his name for me. I don't know for sure if he is a doctor. He looks like a bus conductor or a phlebotomist.

Section 2 Assessment will take place in hospital in Scarborough.

4:00 in the morning. No hot water in the shower. Enjoy!

Still here – wherever - it's Sunday. Felt well enough to go home today, but got the reply: 'No one is going home on Sunday. Wait until a doctor comes on

Monday.' Doctor came on Monday. No change. Fell asleep and missed breakfast. Perhaps as well as I've been eating vacuously all week, I can't get enough food inside me.

The local nut cases are singing Christmas songs to the karaoke. Red Jumper returned. After much hanging about and demanding, I managed to get a bath. It says on the door 'assisted bathroom' but there is no assistance. It has no grab rails and the bath is less than 5 foot long. It's on a timer. Only runs for a short time. You have to ask for everything. Finally, finally, I managed to obtain a hair dryer, but no one has a comb. If I wasn't sane, this place would drive you up the wall.

I keep asking the time. My watch has been stolen. There are no clocks. I think it is about 10:30, so maybe about an hour and a half to Sunday dinner. To be fair, I've enjoyed some of the dinners. Chicken masala was good with sweet corn and then sticky toffee pudding.

I'm dressed like a tramp. My clothes have been stolen. I'm in a borrowed leather jacket and jogging bottoms.

Mentally, I feel stronger. But I'm not right yet. Obviously it would be better if I could recover at home. But there are too many of them here against me. I think the best course of action is to keep myself mentally alert and watch them like a hawk.

It would not surprise me if they did not let me out tomorrow. In a way I don't want them to. It gives me more time to observe them. There have been some acts of kindness. Alpen bars, bag of crisps, even a glass of milk. But there is something going on here and I want to see how they resolve it. I don't want to force the issue.

Every door is still locked, including the fire doors, the laundry room, the storeroom. I can see clothes in there, but I can't get at them.

I suppose the best way to treat it is as an incarceration, like a prison sentence. It sounds a funny thing for me to say, but in a way I'm not that bothered when it ends. I've got a lot of things to do when I get out of here. I know I can cope with this. I am doing. It's mad, but it's a madness that I have grown accustomed to. It will be a very strange day indeed when they do show me the door.

Finally managed to get a bowl of Rice Krispies for breakfast. These little triumphs keep me going. And as you can see, I have now obtained a pen to write with. Winning these little battles does give my brain a lift. Makes it feel better. I'm not convinced that is what it is designed to do, but that is the effect it has.

The list of medications is curious. There must be over a dozen pills, so there's clearly a mind working here. I've seen several doctors, very distinguished looking doctors. We cannot just dismiss them. I think my best policy is to listen to what they say and not challenge them. Obviously a doctor cannot let you out unless he thinks you are well enough to look after yourself. So perhaps engage him in some academic discussion. In which the roles were reversed.

Mental illness is a difficult thing to treat. I have offered to work with him on a paper to examine my case. Have you heard of my psychiatrist, Mr Will at York District Hospital? It would be interesting for the three of us to discuss my case in detail. The problem, of course, is time. Doctor Will did not want to release me from his list but was forced to by pressure from the NHS. Can a way be found around that?

I was weighed and measured today. I have shrunk 2 inches but still weigh 12 stone. The ravages on my body are clear to see and yet I feel strong. I've had to put up with comments about my short stature all my life. But really it is only my legs that are short. They're 2 foot long. If they were 3 foot long, I would be 6 foot tall.

Clearly, there is a lot to be learned in the treatment of mental illness. I think my case is unique. I would like to work with you and the doctors to find a more humane way of treating mental illness.

It is definitely not the case that you treat mental illness kindly. The patient has to fight and fight and fight. It has been extremely distressing at times. I have the bruises to prove it. But as you can imagine, my wife dying after 45 years made me very angry indeed. I needed an outlet for that anger. And you have provided it.

I have researched my first two breakdowns. I'm not a doctor, I'm a planning surveyor. Planning is what I do. And I can see a plan here with me, the guinea pig. My initial thoughts were to expose this scandalous treatment of a mentally ill patient, but I have had time to look at this in the round and think we have a tremendous opportunity to change psychiatry for good.

Clearly some things do need to change. Not many people could take the battering and bruising I have taken. Some other means of releasing that anger needs to be found.

Wild Scottish mountain trails, the wind and the rain lashing your face until you are exhausted. I think exhaustion is the key.

I'm not completely well yet, but I think my mental illness has been blasted out of my mind.

My strength will return with a good bit of nurturing, rest, and relaxation. Unfortunately, I don't have the love of a good woman anymore. That is what I really need now to complete my recovery. May God provide.

Writing this has surprised me. It is cathartic. I feel a great burden has been lifted from my shoulders.

Even in the very rough times when I was being beaten, thrown to the ground, something inside me kept telling me to keep fighting and all will be well. Am I barking up the wrong tree writing to you in this way, Doctor? Do you have a counter argument? All I can say in conclusion is I don't want to waste this.

I have family in Switzerland. They come from a place called Solothurn , so my father told me. I never got the opportunity to visit them myself. My name is STUDER. It would be nice if they could look after me and make me well again. I would love that. They sound like a very nice family. From what my father told me of his father, Felix, he was the black sheep of the family. He was the eldest, but he did something wrong: he sold his share of the family home for a shilling and fled to England. He fathered my father, Victor, and promptly abandoned him, clearing off to London. Yet, despite that, my father idolised him. I would like to know the true story. I could never make any sense of what my father said.

From what I've read, Switzerland is a beautiful country. I would much rather live in Switzerland than England. To be honest, I have never felt particularly English. I don't look English and I do love the mountains of Scotland, which is the nearest I have been to that kind of scenery.

Switzerland is a clean, stable country with very sensible laws. And neutral. They don't go to war. I would be proud to be Swiss. They are a rich country, yes, but they do not flaunt their money like America does. They have common sense: I like their attitude to assisted dying, for example. I must state I have no desire to die. I want to live a long time and re-discover my long lost country. I feel like I have been on a journey of discovery. Names, faces, places glimpsed in a chimera. I thought I might have a gift for languages. But I do not, although I do like languages.

There are so many questions. One of the most beautiful things I like is water from a cool mountain stream. I love the ice and the snow, but I've never been skiing. It seems so fast and dangerous. I do like speed. I was a sprinter as a boy, very fast, 100 yards, 200 yards. I always wondered where that came from. And I do like small, precise things, beautifully made. No, I would not be sad to turn my back on England for the cool, crisp mountains of Switzerland. And into the fresh air.

I did love my Diane. To be fair, I was in a bit of a state when she met me: lonely, drinking too much, never had a girlfriend. She was in a state too, separated from her husband, who had made another woman pregnant; taking Valium like sweets. She was moody, often hit me, but I took it because I was desperate. There was no one else. We stuck together for 45 years because throughout most of those years, one or the other of us was ill. Her dying was like a triple whammy. I was free from her. It was like falling off a cliff. I had no idea where I would land, if I would land. If I would finally wake up and live the life I was meant to do.

I have been abused all my life. My mother had another son called Chris from a previous marriage. He was nothing like me. 6 foot tall, academic: Grammar School, University. My mother ignored all my natural talents and embarked on a scheme to make me follow his example. Her husband, Victor, was her henchman. Unfortunately I am a nice lad and always try to please but I could not do it. They finally told me that Chris had a different father when I was 21. I fled back to Nottingham where I was doing an HND in Building. I did find a job that I liked as a Planning Surveyor. But again, I was at the beck and call of someone: this time it was site managers, wanting materials. All I can say is that I have done the best I could throughout my life. What more can a man do?

So here I am, still sitting at a playroom table trying to work out my life. I have been told that I can appeal against the Section. They have appointed someone called Mark Williams, who is my legal representative, but it will be after Christmas, face to face. They're not giving up on this. It looks like I have more battles to come. What will be the outcome? I do not know. Will I get a break? Will this Mark Williams be any good?

Even after all this time, there are still so many balls up in the air that could land anywhere. Once again I ask myself, is there a purpose in this? Is the Tribunal the only way to sort this out? A Tribunal is legally binding, isn't it? It has the power of the law behind it.

Time not known. Drinking coffee. They have finally returned my warm Mountain Warehouse coat to me, my blue trousers and my left blue sock. I've had to ask for another pen. All I can do is write. There doesn't seem anything I can do to get to sleep. I've been laying on my bed in my borrowed clothes, but I'm warmer now in some of my own clothes. This is the first time I've seen this jacket since I've been here. The first time I've been warm.

Going to the toilet is a constant problem. There is no proper toilet paper, just tissues. My poo is black and dry. I found my other sock tucked into my waistband. I remember I tried it there to stop my trousers coming down. Going to sit in the hall with the inmates. Sweating now.

Today is Monday. The time is 2:52. The weather is 3° C. The cloud base 3 degrees, height 1° left, wind speed not known. Is there any activity? None. How far is it to the next person? I'm going to teach you how to rhyme. What rhymes with sausage in your own language? Shallowaba. There is no one with me now. Another one is back and just plugged something in. I'm writing well. The pen is good. Coffee is good. I keep writing. I enjoy writing.

Different room moved many times in bed. Treatment for COVID.

21st December Darlington Memorial Hospital. Here because I'm feeling sick. Been here 2 days. Doctors to decide now. Name of doctor denied. 7:15 AM Breakfast. 8:00 AM Just me, more than 10 staff keeping watch. COVID. Isolation. Confined to bedroom. Laying on bed, back aches, neck aches, stomach aches. Drinking constantly. No relief. Guards right throughout the night, food horrible and goes right through me. Don't know what day it is. No difference day or night.

More peaceful night. Exercising a bit of control of my mind to create scenarios where I find some pleasure. Looked in the mirror, my face looks peaceful though my body doesn't feel it. Still able to write, I don't know what will happen.

Keeping back ramrod straight. Orange juice and Rice Krispies. Shower. Hot water on back. Some relief.

They call me Granddad now. Someone has just been in saying he is cleaning Granddad's room. He said the time was 10:30.

Crap fish. Chips inedible. Carrots, Orange juice. Back stiff, stomach OK, Shoulder ache. Headache.

I have a chair and a desk. It seems that by this Section 5, they can detain you for as long as they want to. It overrides your human rights. I am stronger. I do like writing. So long as I can write, that is the thing. I will read this again.

Laid on my back with my feet high up the wall for a remarkable length of time. Can't say I noticed much relief from back pain. I have re-read the report a dozen times.

On back again. Legs up the wall as before. Asked for a bath. Denied. Because I have COVID. Apparently. Not. Towels thrown on floor for a shower. Do not want another shower. That seems no end to this, but as George said, 'all things must pass'.

Extraordinary range of food. Sausage rolls, scotch egg, egg sandwich, quiche. Double portions of everything.

I'm going through every song I have written. Better than I have ever before. It's the performance to beat every performance in the world. How long can I keep going?

My main problem tonight is breathing. My reflex breathing is not working. I'm having to take every breath. Back OK. Neck OK. Mind OK. No relief in the shower for this one. I think tomorrow is Christmas Eve. Temperature OK, dressed in pyjamas that are filthy. The entertainment from my mind today has been extraordinary. Really, really funny. Finishing off stories, creating new ones. I have to keep my stomach distended trying to relax when I can.

Well, here's the thing. I'm wide awake. I don't think I've ever been so wide awake. So let's plan.

1. Haircut.

2. Contact Mr Ernest
   (accountant I sent a book to).

3. Contact Wood and Richardson (printer).

4. Research literary agents.

5. Research Publishers.

6. Assemble medical team: psychiatrist, doctor, personal trainer, dietitian.

7. Buy Holiday home in Filey.

8. Clothes - Browns, Personal shopper.

9. Guitar lessons.

10. Singing lessons.

11. Acting lessons.

12. Comedy lessons.

13. Yoga but not in a class.

14. Meditation.

15. Swimming lessons.

Random act of kindness: girl bought me two glasses of milk. She seemed worried about me, which is a first. When I have these breakdowns, I usually make a friend. I think the problem this time is I've been confined to my room so I haven't had the opportunity to make a friend. There was one bloke, but he turned out to be cruel to me in equal parts.

Stomach very upset all night. Bowl of Rice Krispies for breakfast. Sun shining on my face this morning. Stomach just starting to settle. I've just had a horrible dream in which I was in the back seat of a car with the door still open. But it trapped me so that I couldn't breathe. It felt very real. Then I remembered I have been transported in taxis at night. In one, my back was so bad I was laid flat out with my legs above my head while the female guard and the taxi driver chatted up front. Just pyjamas, very cold. Modern taxi electric, I think. Black seats, no glasses, blurred vision.

I have another memory: Darlington Memorial Hospital waiting room. Being pushed round and round on a wheelchair because I couldn't stand sitting in the uncomfortable chairs anymore. Collapsed in the toilet. Two guards shoved me on to a trolley and held me there forcibly. No one took any notice. There was a lot more incidents like that in the same vein. The level of violence and cruelty was off the scale.

Same hospital, coffee shop, Normal. Surreal. Everyone going about their business. Me in agony.

I've just asked for a glass of fruit juice. I do not have any way of telling the time.

3 COVID tests today up my nose. Horrible. Test 1 result not given.

Test 2 negative.

Test 3 looks clear to me. He says it should be alright for tomorrow.

Make demand for bath, clothes, advocate. Waiting. Christmas Day tomorrow.

Cried my eyes out tonight when he gave me my meds, said I wanted to go home. They've broken me. I give up. Someone tapped me on the shoulder and asked if I would like to go back to York tonight. I said 'of course, anytime'. She said she would try and arrange transport. That was a while ago. Games again?

Dressed in new Primark gear. Transport to York promised for 9:00. Time 8:45 in the evening. I'm in Doncaster to be transported to Moss Park, York. Like a prisoner. Locked in the room again. Still treating me like I have COVID. Given sandwiches and a cup of tea. It's the same as the last place. But new.

Survived a difficult night. Thought I was a goner. Too hot, no air. Couldn't breathe. Collapsed on the floor outside my cell door. No sympathy, Opened window for me. Bed too hard, couldn't get comfortable, mouth very very dry. Felt like it was filled with sticks. Dying felt only moments away. Don't know how, I asked for a cup of coffee. Dunked some biscuits in and gradually managed to claw myself back to life. Worst night so far.

This morning I have decided to go on a charm offensive. I couldn't be more pleasant, cooperative, the model patient. It's working. They returned with friendly actions, even bought me a Christmas present. Yet another COVID test. Yet another fail.

Weighed 10.2 stone. I'm not going to mention the appeal. I'll continue with the charm offensive.

Christmas dinner, soup - and pudding, the best bit. Too much. Tasted, OK. Provided a radio. I'm taking exaggerated care of myself. I'm going to play with the radio now. Christmas Day was a day of music, fantastic music on the radio. I've never known such great music, song after song.

It is one in the morning now. My back aches. I'm having a cup of tea. I wanted to shower but no hot water. Got dressed.

Boxing Day 5:00 AM. Asked for electric razor. Breakfast: chocolate. Finally had shower. Feel very strong. Asked to see manager repeatedly. Not turned up yet.

Manager Johnny Long finally turned up. Asked him what possible reason he had for keeping me here, he said it was the Section. A doctor would have to release me from the Section. No doctor was available. I said I wanted release today. He said he could not. He's a young lad. I asked him what salary he was on. He said he was not well paid.

Walking around. Confrontation with big bastard manager, 6 foot 7 inches. Demanded my belongings returned. Returned wallet with money and wedding ring and shoelaces. No phone though. I will continue.

Exercised my right to read the paper in the lounge. Faced them down, including the big bastard manager. I sat as long as I could in the uncomfortable chair and only retreated to my bedroom when my backside could stand it no longer.

Found receipt in my wallet from Asda. They spent £50 of my own money on Primark clothing for me without asking my permission. Had a good chat with one of the nurses called Caroline, Best one so far. She assured me that they would allow me home, possibly on a short visit at first, if I did not antagonise them. She said that Johnny Long and David were good nurses and will help me. I have yet to see evidence of that, but I will let you know.

Not a bad night. 8:00 AM Tuesday 27th December. Had shower; asked for a hair dryer and a comb. And Rice Krispies.

I had better ring my brother because he will be wondering what has happened to me. I can't believe how obstructive they are to me ringing Chris. They finally found his number. Eventually they produced a mobile phone, but it was flat. I tried my own phone, also flat and no money. They eventually put my phone on charge. I started this at 8:00 this morning. It is now 12:00. No progress.

Had a visit from a vicar, or pastor, as he calls himself. Full of platitudes and insincere words, he had the audacity to question me about my wife. I ended up telling him I wouldn't pay him in washers. He soaked it up like a sponge. Tried all day to phone my brother. Their mobile not working, my mobile not working. Did manage to contact the bank, told them my cards had been stolen. They will replace them, but it will take 5 days. I have £120 in cash in my wallet.

I seem to be turning vegetarian. Vegetable meatballs, Veggie lasagna. Very nice. I'll continue with this at home.

Finally got to see the elusive David. Told him that my wife had died on 3rd November and that I had been incarcerated in secure mental hospitals ever since. Told him I needed to send out death certificates urgently and I wanted to do that tomorrow. I told him I needed three to four hours at home and would come back afterwards, if that was what was wanted. Can he guarantee that I could do that? He would not guarantee it. He said he would hand it over to someone else in the morning. Told him the same as I told the vicar: that he was a disgrace to the nursing profession and that I wouldn't pay him in washers. He soaked it up like a sponge. I told him that he should be outraged that I say that to him. He cleared off.

New Year's Eve. Promised by the doctor that I could go home on my own today to do some gardening. Repeated this request throughout the morning. The nurse in charge keeps saying she has to consult with colleagues. Asked her again at 11:00. Request denied. The ON CALL consultant will not release me from the Section so that I can go home and sleep in my own bed. I did not get any sleep last night because the window would not open and it was too warm to sleep.

Tuesday 3rd January: surprise meeting with psychiatrist Brine and his team: Physiotherapists, Assistant Psychologist, Occupational Therapist, Chief Nurse, CPN. It was an interrogation like a Tribunal. I made Brine read out loud my conclusion. He and all the others soaked it up like a sponge. It made no impression on them. I insulted each and every one of them and praised them in turn. No impression.

The CPN wants to see me in the ward on Thursday at 1:30. I said I would see him at home and he refused. Brine would not release me no matter what I said. I asked him to convene a meeting like this once a week to discuss my case. He refused. He thinks he can make me better by keeping me here. I told him that was a load of *******.

Anouska was very bad, quoting that I had sung her my songs, which she should not have done. Betrayed again. I thought she was my friend. None of them are my friends. They're all bastards. Brine said it was a funny way to end the meeting, when I insulted him. He's just a boy, no more than 30 years old. How can he be a consultant at that age?

Consultants should be 50 at least. He knows nothing about my mental illness, knows nothing about breakdowns. Said the term breakdown means different things to different people, yet he sits in judgement of me. He controls my life. I stormed out of the meeting.

Met a nice lady called Abbey, a Methodist. She really did listen to what I had to say. I showed her everything. She even said a prayer with me. I pleaded with her to use her influence on Brine to get me released. She said she would try. I cannot ask more than that. She is coming every Monday. I felt better having talked to Abbey.

Evening meal not delivered as per menu, again. Refused what they offered. They offered an alternative: vegetarian meatballs, which I refused. Had a couple of crap mince pies. That's all I had for tea. Told them to order me a McDonald's. They refused. Then told me to order and pay for it myself. I agreed. But said I could not use my own phone because it has no money on it. They offered me the ward phone, but I said my card does not work. Slammed the door in my face. Made a cup of tea with my own tea bag and went back to my room. Where I am now writing this.

Tried all day to get permission to travel to Acomb Funeral Home to collect Diane's ashes. I was ready with my boots on at 7:00 this morning. I've just taken my boots off, they're not going to allow me to go.

Tried a dozen times to ring Julie last night, right up until midnight. She answered the first time and put the phone down. Each time I rang after that, she was on another line. Rang Chris. He said she doesn't have another line. I did not press it. It was 5:30 in the morning and he didn't sound well. He said he would ring Julie. And find out what's going on, but I've not heard from him.

Chris cannot get hold of Julie. My left hand is painful. They gave me an ice pack, but it didn't work. I told Chris about it. He said he would have a word with them. I used the ice pack all night. No sleep. This morning, 4:30 AM hand not so bad. Asked for a safety, Razor: refused. I normally get up at 5:00 AM.

It's been a fight, but I'm ready to go at 8:30. Been sworn at and thrown to the ground by two big black guards.

Bastards will not let me collect Diane's ashes from the crem again. 7th refusal. Saw Brine. Explained to him in detail why I want to collect my wife's ashes. Made no difference. Talked to CPN on phone. Asked loads of questions, many were personal. Answered them all reasonably. Claimed to understand. But he's the same as the rest.

I sang Diane's memorial service to inmates. They commented on how nice the singing was.

Two black guards assaulted me at 7:30 this morning. Big guard reviewed the CCTV and said there was no evidence I was pushed.

Physio provided a yoga mat and made me use it to demonstrate that I could get on and off it. Brine agreed to schedule my evening tablets for 10:00 so that I can do my relaxation exercises. He wasn't happy about it.

Refused Isobrophen for painful hand: given ice pack again. Wearing unironed pyjamas. They made me a coffee. Watching BBC News 100 years. Very interesting. Guard says I was upset, that's why he wouldn't give me the iron and the ironing board. He looks Welsh, but I've never seen him before. Another long night, no sleep.

Prepared three complaints this morning at 2:30 AM, 7:35 AM and 9:10 AM. Asked at the office door if Brine had a pigeon hole. He appeared behind me. I showed him the complaints, walked into the office, made him read them. No response. Stood my ground. Forced out of the office. Meeting went on until 10:00, door still closed. Knocked and kicked;

door not opened. When door did open, I stood in office and demanded to know when I can go home. Manhandled; fell to the floor in the office. Manhandled out of the office on an inflatable slide sheet. Disgraceful. Like Victorian nuthouse, I've never been so insulted in all my life and I have had a lot of insults from hospitals. It was the big guard that evicted me. Brine was still on the phone. I think he's chicken.

Confronted Brine in the office again. Kept voice low. Asked when I would be allowed home, he said soon. I refused to move from the office. Manhandled again, fell to the floor, again in the doorway. Manhandled out of the office on an inflatable slide sheet again. I shouted at Brine: 'Are you pleased with this? You should be struck off. I will make it my business to get you struck off.' No response from Brine; still on the phone.

Run out of PG tips, pyramid tea bags. Paid one of the nurses £5 to buy some.

11:00 PM Made tea with lukewarm water. Mug of milk. David on duty: talked to him, trying to make friends with the wardens so that they would not ill treat me tonight.

Woke up this morning on the floor, but quite comfortable. I sleep fully clothed. It's the only way to keep warm. They gave me a sleeping tablet last night and that's what knocked me out.

Big bowl of Bran Flakes and two cups of tea. Feel alright; better than I have done for a long time. The time is 4:10 AM.

Refused permission to go to church on Sunday, January 8th. Ian Till, vicar, is coming to see me at the hospital on Wednesday 2:00.

Ordered a McDonald's for 12:00. It came at 12:30. OK, edible; milkshake - best bit. Tuna pasta bake for tea, lemon sponge and custard Time 3:50 PM.

Six

COMPLAINTS

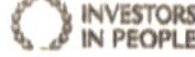

NHS
Tees, Esk and Wear Valleys
NHS Foundation Trust

Complaints Department
Flatts Lane Centre
Normanby
Middlesbrough
TS6 0SZ

Tel: 0800 052 0219
Website: www.tewv.nhs.uk

Ref: 49089/GR

23rd January 2022

Private & Confidential
Mr P Studer
Moorcroft
Foss Park Hospital
York

Dear Mr Studer

Thank you for your email regarding your complaint which was received on 28th December 2022. I was sorry to read your concerns about your stay on Moorcroft Ward as an inpatient in Foss Park Hospital, York.

As part of my investigation we asked Moorcroft ward to provide a statement regarding your concerns and this is their response:-

1. **Mr Studer would like to know why at present that he is not allowed any leave from the ward?**

    Moorcroft Ward confirm that due to the Christmas Period, unfortunately they did not have a consultant available to review your section 17 leave up until the 28th December 2022 and the team apologise for this. The team have confirmed that they prioritised your request and a covering consultant agreed to give you 2 hours section 17 leave in the local area escorted by staff members from the ward and this was facilitated on the 28th December 2022. The Trust apologise for the lack of consultants available at this time.

73

2. Mr Studer states that he has had 10 items stolen whilst an inpatient, but these items are not listed on the letter, does the ward have a list of the items and their value?

   The ward has confirmed that you have been transferred to a number of different wards during your recovery both within our trust and Darlington Memorial Acute Hospital. From the electronic record we can confirm that you were initially admitted to Rowan Lea Ward Scarborough, then Moorcroft, then Cedar Ward PICU, then Bedale Ward PICU, back to Cedar Ward PICU, then Darlington Memorial Hospital, then to Cedar Ward PICU and finally back to Moorcroft Ward.

   PALS understand that you have provided the ward with items that you believe are missing during your admission to the various wards. From the investigation we can confirm that the following items were given to you when you were transferred back from Cedar Ward PICU which were on your list, which were your wedding ring, shoelaces and wallet with £75 pounds which included your debit card and driving licence. The ward has also confirmed that staff members contacted both Cedar Ward and Bedale Ward to try and locate your other items and both wards have confirmed that they do not have your possessions.

3. Mr Studer states that there is no hot water available for a shower early on a morning please can you confirm if there are problems with the water system on the ward?

   We asked Moorcroft ward to provide a statement regarding your concerns and the ward checked your shower and noted that hot water was available for you.

4. Mr Struder states that he is not being well treated by staff whilst residing on the ward.

   We understand that you were transferred from Cedar Ward PICU while you had covid–19 and that you wanted to wash your clothes on the morning of the 28th December 2022. As Moorcroft's laundry room is off the main ward, due to you having Covid-19 and due to your compliance of mask wearing being variable as there were other patients clothing being stored in the laundry room it was advised that the ward staff would wash your laundry. Staff brought you an iron and ironing board on so that you could iron your clothes after they were washed, and you were able to wash your own clothes following your isolation period which ended on 29th December 2022.

5. Mr Studer states that he is not being well treated by staff whilst residing on the ward.

   The Trust apologise if you feel that you are not being treat well by staff whilst residing on the ward. From the electronic records it is documented that you were transferred to Moorcroft ward from Rowan Lea Ward, Scarborough as you were acutely unwell and the team used restraint and Rapid Tranquilisation due to the risk to others and staff members can confirm that the Trust policies have been followed at all times.

   We understand that the ward has tried to be creative and prioritise your requests to support your recovery since being transferred back to Moorcroft Ward which has been difficult due to it being over the Christmas period.

74

I hope you feel that the concerns you have identified have been given serious consideration and responded to accordingly.

If I can be of any further assistance, please do not hesitate to contact the Patient Advice and Liaison Service.

Yours sincerely

PALS Officer

80

75

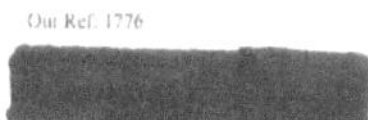

Mr P Studer
Moorcroft Ward
Foss Park Hospital Haxby Road
York
YO31 8TA

Our Ref: 1776

15th February 2023

Dear Mr Studer,

Re: Your Mental Health Matter

We write to confirm that following your Tribunal on the 8th February 2023 the panel chose to not discharge you from your section.

The reasons as to why the Tribunal panel decided your case in that way are set out fully in the enclosed Tribunal Decision.

Having reviewed the decision in detail, ▮▮▮▮▮▮ does not feel that there are grounds to appeal or set aside the order made. As such, we would therefore advise that you are next eligible to appeal to the First Tier Tribunal in the event that your section is renewed for a further 6-month period.

We again can reassure you that your legal costs will be met in full by the Legal Aid Agency. Once those costs have been paid, your file will be closed and safely stored at our office for a period of 6 years, after which it will be securely destroyed.

Yours sincerely,

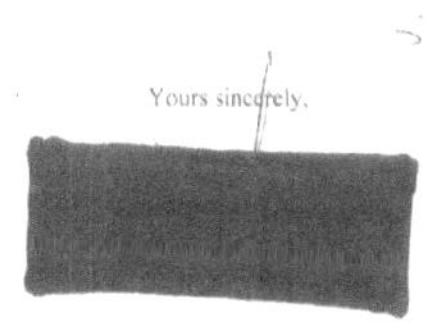

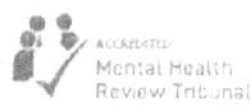

3. Non-RPP
S.3, S.37
(S.47, S.48)
or equivalent

The First-tier Tribunal
(Health, Education and Social Care Chamber)
Mental Health

Mental Health Act 1983 (as amended)
The Tribunal Procedure (First-tier Tribunal) (Health, Education and Social Care Chamber) Rules 2008

Case Number: ▇▇▇▇▇▇
Date of Patient Application: 18/12/2022

Patient: Phillip Studer (born 08/10/1952)

A patient now liable to be detained under Section 3 of the Act

Responsible Authority: Tees, Esk and Wear Valleys NHS Foundation Trust
Hospital: Foss Park Hospital

Before

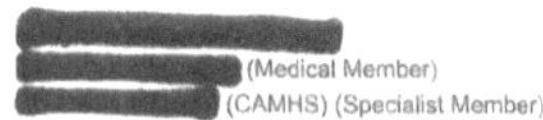

▇▇▇▇▇▇ (Medical Member)
▇▇▇▇▇▇ (CAMHS) (Specialist Member)

Sitting at Foss Park Hospital on 8 February 2023

Decision

The patient shall not be discharged from liability to be detained.

Recommendation(s) pursuant to section 72(3) & (3A)

The tribunal does not make a recommendation.

Representation
Patient: ▇▇▇▇▇▇
Responsible Authority: Not represented.

Attendance by Patient at the remote hearing
The Patient did not attend the hearing

Pre-Hearing Medical Examination of the Patient
A pre-hearing examination of the patient was not indicated under the Rules.

Sept 2021 V

82

<u>Announcement of Decision</u>

The decision was announced at the end of the hearing.

<u>The Tribunal considered</u>

Oral evidence from ▓▓▓▓▓▓▓▓▓▓▓▓▓▓ and ▓▓▓▓▓▓▓
Written evidence from ▓▓▓▓▓▓▓▓▓▓▓▓ and ▓▓▓▓
Other material, namely Responsible Authority's Statement of Information.

<u>Jurisdiction, Preliminary and Procedural Matters</u>

1. The tribunal is satisfied that it has jurisdiction to consider this application
2. The patient's solicitor made application to be appointed under rule 11(7)(b) which was granted

<u>Grounds for the Decision</u>

1. The tribunal is satisfied that the patient is suffering from mental disorder or from mental disorder of a nature or degree which makes it appropriate for the patient to be liable to be detained in a hospital for medical treatment.
2. The tribunal is satisfied that it is necessary for the health or safety of the patient or for the protection of other persons that the patient should receive such treatment.
3. The tribunal is satisfied that appropriate medical treatment is available for the patient.
4. The tribunal does not consider that it is appropriate to discharge the patient under its discretionary powers.

<u>Reasons</u>

1. The patient's factual and psychiatric history was not challenged, is well known to the parties and so it is not necessary to recite it here verbatim.

2. The patient's wife passed away in November 2022 and prior to that he had experienced 6 weeks of poor sleep. After her death he became agitated and disinhibited and began acting in a bizarre manner. He planned to sell his car, travel to Switzerland and made an offer to purchase a new house. He saw his GP who advised antipsychotic medications which he declined to take believing them to be expired and poisonous. He self-presented to Cross Lane Hospital where he was reviewed by the Crisis Team and admitted. At that time he was found to be irritable, angry and grandiose.

3. Post admission he was transferred to Foss Park Hospital on 18/11/2022 where he refused to accept oral medications including oral rapid tranquilisation. He presented as agitated, notified the police he had been kidnapped and made requests to leave the ward. He required repeated IM medications due to escalating behaviours, frequently placing himself on the ground, throwing furniture, and invading others personal space. He was transferred to the PICU where he similarly presented. He refused food/fluids and oral medications, requiring seclusion on 25/11/2022. When his mental health improved he was transferred back to Foss Park Hospital on 24/12/2022.

4. The RC's diagnosis is one of bipolar affective disorder, current episode manic with psychotic symptoms.

5. The team agree that the patient could not be managed outside of a hospital setting and the patient has no capacity to consent to informal treatment.

Sept 2021 V

83

78

6. Appropriate medical treatment is available in the form of medication, a safe and structured environment, medical supervision and skilled nursing care and supervision.

7. Were the patient to not receive this treatment his mental state would deteriorate further and he would be exposed to all three areas of risk.

8. The patient did not give evidence but was represented by his solicitor  who was acting in his best interests.

9. There was no significant challenge to the written evidence presented by the treating team and no further evidence adduced which might undermine it. We can therefore contract these reasons and the route to our findings to reflect the absence of challenge.

10. In the circumstances, looking at the evidence in the round, we find the evidence of the treating team persuasive in relation to not only the description of the disorder, but also the risks associated with the removal of the order and in relation to the provision of appropriate treatment. The patient presents with risks to himself through self-neglect, self-harm, and through his behaviours. There are also risks to others through his physical and verbal aggression.

11. We therefore accept the evidence from the treating team and agree that the order should not be discharged.

12. We do not exercise our discretionary power to discharge for the reasons set out above.

Judge 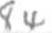
Date: 8/2/23

Notice

A person seeking permission to appeal must make a written application to the tribunal for permission to appeal. An application for permission must:

    a. identify the decision of the tribunal to which it relates;

    b. identify the alleged error or errors of law in the decision; and

    c. state the result the party making the application is seeking.

An application for permission must be sent or delivered to the tribunal so that it is received no later than 28 days after the latest of the dates that the tribunal sends to the person making the application:

    a. written reasons for the decision;

    b. notification of amended reasons for, or correction of, the decision following a review; or

    c. notification that an application for the decision to be set aside has been unsuccessful. (Note: This date only applies if the application for the decision to be set aside was made within the initial 28-day time limit, or any extension of that time previously granted by the tribunal.)

If the person seeking permission to appeal sends or delivers the application to the tribunal later than the time required then:

    a. the application must include a request that the tribunal extends the time limit under Rule 5(3)(a), and give the reason(s) why the application was not provided in time; and

Sept 2021 v

MHA 1983 Section 17 Leave of Absence

Tees, Esk and Wear Valleys **NHS**
NHS Foundation Trust

| Patient Name | Phillip Studer (Preferred name Paul) | Paris ID | 984548 | Section | 3 | Ward | Moor Croft | RC | Dr |

I, the Responsible Clinician for the above named patient, authorise leave of absence as detailed below

Regular/Specified Leave

From		To		Destination and Reason (please include number of hours, occasions, weekly or daily if appropriate)	Escorted? Yes / No	Accompanied? Yes / No	By Whom	Conditions of Leave or Instructions and observations for risk management if accompanied
Date	Time	Date	Time					
07/02/2023	12.35	25/02/2023	23.59	To York Hospital facilities as needed for a frequency and duration dictated by clinical need	Yes	No	Clinical staff of any grade	Escorting staff to be familiar with Paul's current safety plan prior to periods of leave
07/02/2023	12.35	28/02/2023	23.59	For planned therapeutic leave within the local York area for up to a total maximum of 4 hours per day. The precise location of any period of leave will be agreed between the MDT staff and Paul prior to any period of leave.	Yes	No	At least one member of clinical staff of any grade	All leave is at the discretion of the nurse-in-charge and **may be denied** if there are concerns regarding Paul's mental state (eg aggression/hostility) and/or risk assessment at the point of leave.

The conditions of the above leave are that the patient returns to hospital at the time/date stated, agrees to take medication prescribed, is in contact with his/her Care Coordinator, attends CPA reviews/ward rounds where appropriate, escorted/unescorted (please specify by whom ie numbers, level of qualification, gender etc)

Long Term Leave (end date cannot exceed expiry date of section)

From	To	Destination and Reason	Conditions of longer term leave eg to remain in the custody of staff of X care home or hospital

For sections 3/37/45A/47/48: I have considered the use of Supervised Community Treatment and concluded that it is not appropriate at this time and I have fully recorded my reasons for my decision in the patient's Care Record

RC signature   Date   07/02/2023   Accompanying Person Signature (Where relevant)

Patient signature   Date   Date

(Or reason for absence of signature eg unable, refused)

Please ensure a copy is this form is given to relevant people including the patient, accompanying person, carer, casenotes, community staff – original to MHA Dept

MHA 1983 Section 17 Leave of Absence

Tees, Esk and Wear Valleys **NHS**
NHS Foundation Trust

| Patient Name | Phillip Studer (Preferred name Paul) | Paris ID | 984548 | Section | 3 | Ward | Moor Croft | RC | Dr[redacted] |

I, the Responsible Clinician for the above named patient, authorise leave of absence as detailed below

Regular/Specified Leave

From		To		Destination and Reason (please include number of hours, occasions, weekly or daily if appropriate)	Escorted? Yes / No	Accompanied? Yes / No	By Whom	Conditions of Leave or Instructions and observations for risk management if accompanied
Date	Time	Date	Time					
14/02/ 2023	09.25	28/02/ 2023	23.59	To York Hospital facilities as needed for a frequency and duration dictated by clinical need.	Yes	No	Clinical staff of any grade	Escorting staff to be familiar with Paul's current safety plan prior to periods of leave.
14/02/ 2023	09.25	28/02/ 2023	23.59	For planned therapeutic leave within the local York area for up to a total maximum of 3 hours per day. The precise location of any period of leave will be agreed between the MDT staff and Paul prior to any period of leave.	No	No	-	All leave is at the discretion of the nurse-in-charge and may be denied if there are concerns regarding Paul's mental state (eg aggression/hostility) and/or risk assessment at the point of leave.

The conditions of the above leave are: that the patient returns to hospital at the time/date stated, agrees to take medication prescribed, is in contact with his/her Care Coordinator, attends CPA reviews/ward rounds where appropriate, escorted/unescorted (please specify by whom ie numbers, level of qualification, gender etc)

Long Term Leave (end date cannot exceed expiry date of section)

From	To	Destination and Reason	Conditions of longer term leave eg to remain in the custody of staff of X care home or hospital

For sections 3/37/45A/47/48: I have considered the use of Supervised Community Treatment and concluded that it is not appropriate at this time and I have fully recorded my reasons for my decision in the patient's Care Record

RC signature [redacted]   Date 14/02/2023   Accompanying Person Signature (Where relevant)

Patient signature   Date   Date

(Or reason for absence of signature eg unable, refused)

Please ensure a copy is this form is given to relevant people including the patient, accompanying person, carer, casenotes, community staff – original to MHA Dept

Tees, Esk and Wear Valleys **NHS**
NHS Foundation Trust

Date: 24 / 01 / 20 23

The following change to your prescribed medication is being made:

> RISPERADONE reduced to 500 micrograms
> twice daily – this is being withdrawn
> QUETIAPINE has been restarted – 50mg at night

Because:

> we are changing your treatment back to
> Quetiapine as this was helpful for you over
> the last 10 years.
>
> Dont Shave tommorrow

If you have any questions regarding this change you will be able to speak
with a ward doctor or pharmacist.

82

OFFICIAL COMPLAINT

DATE & TIME

Monday 16 January 2023 10:19pm

SUBJECT

Physical assault – again

MAIN PERPETRATOR

Clive

DIARY OF EVENTS

I have been complaining all day that the two television sets were being dominated by the women and I was not able to watch TV. I have nothing against women. They have the freedom to watch whatever they want to watch. My point is that I was not able to watch the TV I wanted to because they were monopolising both TV sets. They did it yesterday all day. And I was not able to watch any TV at all yesterday either.

I went to the office to see if they could do anything about it, but there was no one there. The office was in darkness. I waited outside the office door like a guard from 9:15 PM to 10:00 PM. Most of this time,

2 guards were mopping the floor excessively. I verbally abused them, called them all the names under the sun to try and get them to sort out my TV problem. They verbally abused me back then disappeared. I don't know where they went.

A female guard dressed in black appeared. But took no notice of me. I did not abuse her. A female guard in blue apparel asked me what was the problem. I told her. She told me to move away from the office door and I refused. I did not abuse her.

Clive pressed his alarm to summon help, but he didn't need it. He manhandled me away from the door, threw me face down on the floor, stepped over me into the office. And bang the office door on my feet. He did this three times. None of the others were involved in the abuse, only Clive.

I remained on the floor, face down, spread-eagled for 15 minutes. It was very uncomfortable. I had difficulty in breathing. I thought my glasses were broken, but they seem to be OK.

I have been on the receiving end of this physical abuse from Clive several times before. The man is dangerous. He should be sacked. God knows what he would have done if I had been a woman. After 15 minutes spread-eagled, face down on the floor, I got up with great difficulty and examined myself for damage. There was none, fortunately. I'm a tough bloke, but no thanks to Clive. I went back to my room and examined myself more closely in the mirror. There was a mark on my face from my glasses where they had pressed in the hard wooden floors. Martin, one of the patients is a witness to Clive's latest violence against me, but if he doesn't want to testify, leave him alone; he is a nice lad. He was just playing Scrabble with a guard who was not involved.

I sat down to write this official complaint, which I finished at 10:25 PM.

Three months of laying on my bed in six mental hospitals has atrophied the muscles in my back so that now I walk like an old man. No attempt has been made to give me exercise. They do that in prison. This regime is harsher than in prison.

Paul Studer

Signature of the patient.

OFFICIAL COMPLAINT

DATE & TIME

Friday 6 January 2023 5:45pm

SUBJECT

Evening Meal

DIARY OF EVENTS

No menu for main evening meal. Warned them that I was not eating a crap substitute scratch meal as I have done before. Told them to get me a proper vegetarian meal from the other ward.

5:10 PM Crap food served and I would not eat it. Waited 45 minutes at the counter. Shutters broughtdown. I banged on office door to say I have not had an evening meal. The nurse told me that they had offered it to me but that I would not eat it. I told them I'm not eating that crap and that they should get me a meal from the other ward. The nurse told me it was just the same on the other ward. So I told them to order me a McDonald's. She said I would have to pay for it myself. I refused.

She said there was nothing she could do. And I told her she will not get away with this.

The time is now 5:40 PM. I still have not had my main evening meal. I am submitting this official complaint to the office. We will see what happens.

Paul Studer

Signature of the patient.

OFFICIAL COMPLAINT

DATE & TIME

Tuesday 10 January 2023 1:50pm

SUBJECT

Property lost by staff

MAIN PERPETRATOR

Clive

DIARY OF EVENTS

White shirt lost by Clive in laundry. He denies it, but I remember giving him the shirt with two towels this morning at 5:00 AM when I got up. I have only got 3 shirts. I wanted to wear the white one tomorrow morning.

He threw me out of the office and slammed the door in my face, saying: 'Don't ever accuse me of anything, mister. Ever.' He repeated it and slammed the kitchen door in my face as well.

Paul Studer

Signature of the patient.

OFFICIAL COMPLAINT

DATE & TIME

Tuesday 10 January 2023 7:15am

SUBJECT

Physical assault – again

MAIN PERPETRATOR

Clive

DIARY OF EVENTS

Reported to the office that I was ready to go home. My car was thought to be stolen. I must report it to the police. But I cannot until I have physically checked it. Refused permission to go home. Clive pushed me out of the office again and slammed the door in my face again.

My brother had been sent a parking ticket for my car being parked on a double yellow line. But I was in hospital, so the car should have still been in my garage. So I presumed it had obviously been stolen.

(However, when I later checked in the garage, the car was still there.)

Paul Studer

Signature of the patient.

OFFICIAL COMPLAINT

DATE & TIME

Tuesday 10 January 2023 8:15am

SUBJECT

Door slammed in my face

DIARY OF EVENTS

Leah slammed the office door in my face when I demanded to go home to see to my stolen car and report it to police. Clive did the same thing last night. This is not acceptable behaviour.

They seem to think that my missing white shirt is more important than my missing car. They must be mad.

Paul Studer

Signature of the patient.

OFFICIAL COMPLAINT

DATE & TIME

Tuesday 10 January 2023 11:05am

SUBJECT

Physical assault – again

MAIN PERPETRATOR

Manager, Johnny Long

DIARY OF EVENTS

Refused permission to go home today despite my car being stolen. Johnny Long has not read my official complaints. He says I gave my car to my neighbour. I did when I was having a breakdown, immediately after my wife died. The neighbour he refers to is Peter. He was embarrassed at the gift and did not accept it.

So, my car is locked in my garage and my keys are in your safe. Except my brother Chris has a parking ticket for my car being parked on a double yellow line somewhere last week, which is impossible as I was incarcerated in here. So the only potential explanation is that my car has been stolen. Hence the need to report it to the police. But I can't report it until I have checked the garage to see if it is still there.

I was ready to do this at 4:00 this morning, but Clive refused me permission to call a taxi home. He slammed the office door in my face twice. Manager Johnny Long also slammed the office door in my face. This is disgraceful behaviour by two NHS employees who should be sacked. I insist I go home today to see to my car and report it to the police

I also need to retrieve my dead wife Diane's ashes from the crematorium. I also want to go to the Co-op to ask them who gave them permission to cremate my wife, since I did not. I was Sectioned.

A crime has been committed here which also needs to be reported to the police. I can't think of anything more serious, other than murder. You can't kill a dead body, but cremating it is the nearest thing to it. These crimes need to be reported to the police with the utmost urgency. Any delay could tamper with the evidence. Manager Johnny Long is guilty of obstructing Police and should be arrested, as should

Clive. I don't want to see either of them on this ward again.

Paul Studer

Signature of the patient.

Summary of discussion with ████████ and ██████ (09/01/23). (SOCIAL WORKER)

- There is currently an outbreak of a diarrhoea and vomiting infection on Moor Croft. The Trust's infection control team have advised that **no patient has leave** from the hospital until the ward reopens following the infection.
- At this time (Monday 9th January 2023 morning), we do not expect the ward to reopen until Wednesday **at the earliest.** This will be reviewed on a daily basis.
- Leave (requests and conditions) for each patient is reviewed daily by the multidisciplinary team. Your leave is considered and reviewed by the team daily.
- For any detained (sectioned) patient all leave requests will be reviewed prior to the patient leaving the ward. If the nurse-in-charge or another team member has concerns regarding a patient's mental state or behaviour at the time of them going out then the leave request **may be denied** and the patient will not be allowed out, even if there are prior arrangements in place.
- Behaviours which may raise concern leading to refusal of leave:
  - Aggression: verbal eg shouting, hostile or confrontational words or tone of voice; physical eg behaviours intended to intimidate – standing too close to others/invading personal space, blocking doorways, pushing etc
  - Agitation: signs of increased arousal eg increased pacing, raised voice, breathing more quickly
  - Losing temper easily/quickly

9b

OFFICIAL COMPLAINT

DATE & TIME

Friday 6 January 2023   7:35am

SUBJECT

Refusal of Leave

DIARY OF EVENTS

Shaved, brushed teeth, Breakfast of Rice Krispies and my own tea. Did relaxation exercises, showered, washed hair, dressed in best clothes, blow dried hair and put on best boots. Ready to collect my dead wife Diane's ashes from the crematorium for the 7th morning in a row of asking. Why is there not a taxi ready and waiting to take me there for 8:00 this morning?

Diane's ashes have been buried in the ground at the crematorium, but nobody told me.

Paul Studer

Signature of patient

THE FIRST

BREAKDOWN

Seven

My first breakdown was triggered by being made redundant. I had worked for Shepherd Construction for 25 years: 4 as an Estimator and 21 as a Planning Surveyor. I didn't like estimating, but I did like planning. I fully expected to be a Planner until I retired. I loved the job.

My job was to draw up the construction programme, schedule materials, set targets and measure the bonus. No other building company employed planning surveyors, so even if I felt like leaving, there was nowhere else I could go. I would have to become a site manager, which I didn't want to do.

Up until this point, all my jobs had made money. But the job I was put on last was losing money, about half a million pounds. It was a building society in Harrogate. Before the job started I had a look through the Bill of Quantities and there were mistakes all over the place. I did a few calculations based on my experience of estimating and calculated that the job would lose half a million. I went to see the Area Manager and tried to explain my findings. I said we should send it back, say we had made a mistake and we're withdrawing our tender. When I was in estimating, I remember doing that on one job. But the Area Manager would not hear of it this time.

So when the Quantity Surveyors' monthly valuation showed a half a millionpound loss, I was not surprised. The Area Manager got the sack. A new Area Manager called Jack was appointed. He told me to: 'find the money or heads will roll'.

Things did not improve. In fact, they got worse. Jack ordered me to his office and repeated his threat, adding: 'your head will roll'.

I had never been under so much pressure. I started to shake. My stomach hurt. I couldn't sleep. Diane made me an appointment with the doctor I had a good doctor that I had known for years. I remember when he started as a young lad. He asked me: 'Is it worth it? Why don't you just leave and get another job?' But it wasn't that easy. I wanted to remain a Planner, but if I left I would have to give that up and become a site manager. And I didn't want to do that. The doctor gave me some Valium, which helped. Nothing changed, but I didn't care as much thanks to my little yellow pills.

I had a phone call one morning from Jack saying he wanted to see me in his office immediately. I told the site manager that Jack wanted to see me. And he began saying: 'It's been a pleasure working with you'. He wished me well in my future career. I didn't know what he was talking about. I knocked on Jack's door and, without any preamble, he said: 'I'm making you redundant. Clean your desk and go. Don't touch anything'.

I started to protest, but Jack wasn't listening. He stood up and held out his hand. I didn't shake it. I stormed out and slammed the door. That was the end of my 25 year career with Shepherd Construction. I drove home. I think it was about 10:00 in the morning. Diane knew something was wrong as soon as she saw my face. I said: 'I've been made redundant', and she burst into tears. I wish I could have done that too, but I was too angry.

They gave me £14,000 of redundancy money. And this was in 1994, when that represented a lot of money. I should have taken some time off, had a holiday, work out what to do with the rest of my life, but I needed a job. I needed to prove to them and to myself that I was not useless, that I was a valued employee.

As luck would have it, there was an advert in the York Press for an Estimator with a small building firm in Strensall. I hadn't done any estimating for 20 years, but I had kept my estimating notes. I reckoned I could do it. I replied to the advert and had a successful interview and got the job. It was just an act. I lied to them, making out I was an Estimator, ignoring the fact that I had been a Planner for 20 years. I'm very good at interviews. I have a bit of a silver tongue when I care to use it.

They didn't check my references. If they had, they would have found out I was lying. But the most amazing thing was that I was able to slot back in as an Estimator as if I had never been away. I don't like estimating, but I could do it. The job wasn't the problem. The problem was I couldn't come to terms with being made redundant. I was like a wounded animal licking my wounds. I was operating as two people, an Estimator and a redundant Planner.

I won a job, quite a big job, at Menwith Hill. They were very pleased, but my mind was in turmoil. I had to get away from this terrible life I was leading. I planned my escape very carefully. There were some things I didn't want to lose, especially my Estimating and Planning notes. I went to a supermarket in town and bought a cardboard box, filled it and took it to Parcel Force. I addressed it to my mother and father's house.

Diane used to go shopping on Tuesdays with her mother and father. I made up some excuse at work, went home, packed a bag and drove to the Park and Ride. I left a note on the kitchen worktop saying:

'Sorry flower, I can't take anymore. I have to get away. The car is in the Park and Ride car park; keys in the glove compartment.'

I caught the bus to the train station and bought a one way ticket to Kings Cross, London. When I got to London. I walked out of the station and to the road opposite. I kept walking until I came to a hotel. I booked a room for a couple of nights. My mind was buzzing with things I wanted to do:

1. Find a recording studio.
2. Buy a suit.
3. Buy some contact lenses.
4. Have a haircut.
5. Buy a computer.
6. Buy a guitar.
7. Buy a keyboard.
8. Get a passport.

And many more.

I had a taxi and kept him all week, giving him £100 when he asked for it. I had withdrawn £7000 from our building society account, but they would only let me have

£2000 in cash. The rest was in a cheque. I went to a travel agent and bought £5000 worth of dollar travelling cheques. I had an ambition to go to America. I bought a chalkboard from Rymans, chalking on it what I wanted to do; rubbed it out and wrote another note.

The taxi took me to the Passport Office. I filled in the form and forged my neighbour, Paul's signature as a witness. But they found me out. They rang Paul's phone number and spoke to him. No, he wasn't in London. No, he had not signed the form. They gave me a ticking off. I thought they were going to send for the police but they let me off. Normally I would be horrified by such a telling off, but 'The Other Person' wasn't bothered. He thought it was great fun.

I should explain I was operating as two people, my normal self and The Other Person, who did all these crazy things. The Other Person had also started smoking. I had never smoked. I asked the receptionist at the hotel if there was a church nearby. She said there was one at the back of the hotel. This was 9:00 AM on a Sunday. I went to church at 10:00. It was C of E. Partway through the service, I burst into tears. Great big sobs. I couldn't stop them. After the service, they took me into a room where they were serving tea and coffee. They were very nice to me. They wanted to know what was the matter. I tried to tell them, but I couldn't get my words out. I kept on sobbing.

I noticed a lot of black people filing into the church and asked if there was another service. They said: 'yes, it's a gospel service'. I said I would like to go to that and they said I could, that they would have a word with them. I wanted to sit at the back, but they led me halfway down the aisle on an end seat. The singing was fantastic. Such voices. I had never heard such singing before.

I should explain. All my senses were heightened. Everything was fantastic, the best I had ever known. After the service, I said that I had written a song that I would like them to sing. It's called Freedom. I sang it to them and they liked it and said I would have to come to their rehearsal next week. But I never made it.

I couldn't stay at the hotel for very long. It was too expensive. I bought a copy of the London Evening Standard. There was a block of flats in Chelsea with vacancies. I went to see them. Yes, they had a bedsit. It would cost £2500 for a month. I rented the flat.

I walked into Austin Reed and bought two suits. They took my travellers cheques as payment. No problem. But the suits would have to be altered. I have short arms and legs. It would take a week. I never made it.

I walked into an opticians and made an appointment to have my eyes tested for contact lenses. But I never made it.

I was not sleeping. I was awake all night. About midnight, I decided to go to Abbey Road Studios. I flagged down a taxi and asked him to take me there. I walked into the studio and said I would like to record a song. The guard asked if I had an appointment. I told him I didn't. He told me to wait there and he'd see what he could do. He picked up the phone. I lit a cigarette. But The Other Person was impatient. He started walking down the corridor towards the studios. The guard jumped on me and pinned me to the ground. He called the police.

The police were very good. I'm a short bloke. The guard was a big bloke. Police criticised the guard, saying he was supposed to use reasonable force when making an arrest. He had flattened me. It was like being at the bottom of the ruck in rugby.

One of the policeman was black. I told him about the amazing gospel service I'd been to. He said he would look it up, that it sounded good. The police wished me well and off they went. I flagged down a taxi and asked the driver to take me to the Air Studios.

As we pulled up outside the studios. I said: 'They're not going to like this'. I got out of the cab, turned left and let myself into the studio by a side door. It was an old church. It still had the pews around the walls. I walked down to the centre of the church where the microphones were and shouted: 'Turn on the microphone'. When I was in Abbey Road, pinned to the floor by the guard, a song had started to form in my mind.

'I love black people, Yeah, I love black people. Won't you help me, black people, body and soul. Well'.

This was the song I started singing. Two people came and tried to reason with me, but I wouldn't listen. I kept saying: 'Turn on the microphone'. They rang the police and this time they did arrest me and put me in the back of a police van. I would not stop singing. At the station, they sat me in front of a duty Sergeant who tried to ask me questions, but I wouldn't stop singing. A woman police officer twisted my ear. Very painful. But it didn't stop me singing. They put me in a cell, still singing. I can't remember how long I was in the cell. It seemed a long time, but was probably only a few hours.

A prison visitor came to see me. She was very good. She quickly realised that I was having some sort of mental breakdown and needed to be admitted to hospital. Because the address of my flat was in Chelsea, I was taken to a private hospital in Chelsea. They were amazing. They gave me a drug that knocked me out cold. The first time I had slept since coming to London. But I wasn't there long. They soon packed me off to the Chelsea and Westminster Hospital.

They rang Diane. She came to see me. Poor girl. Her husband was a nutter. She didn't know him anymore. But she stuck to me and saw me through. I don't know what I would have done without her.

Eight

In hospital, my mind was in turmoil. I felt like I was in danger of losing control, and if that happened, I would be a vegetable. They diagnosed me with hypomania and gave me drugs, but they didn't seem to have any effect. I was awake day and night. I couldn't keep still. I walked down the corridor, down the steps, around the ground floor corridor, into the courtyard garden, walked around the courtyard garden and retraced my steps back to my bedroom. On the way, I collected a cup of water. All night I kept up the walking until my legs started to give way. I got down on my hands and knees and banged my forehead on the concrete floor. I needed the pain to keep me in the here and now.

In the morning, Diane came to see me and I walked around the park. I was like that for two weeks before my mind started to calm down. Altogether, I was in hospital for 10 weeks. They discharged me into the care of Bootham Park Hospital in York. I was a day patient at Moorlyn. Moorlyn specialised in occupational therapy. Painting was my favourite and yoga. They also did relaxation classes.

Gradually my mind started to slow down, but there was always a part of me that was moving, usually my foot. I still have that. We played badminton. I enjoyed that. I used to play at school and was quite good. I enjoyed my time at Moorlyn. Unfortunately, it is closed now. Replaced by Moss Park, which is nowhere near as good.

I was off work for about a year. Money was tight. We survived on benefits of £75 a week and dipped into our savings. I needed to get back to work. There was an advert in the York Press for a Planner at a construction firm in Ilkley, and as luck would have it, I knew one of the Project Managers there. I got the job.

It went well at first. They liked my programmes. That was all they wanted me to do, draw up programmes. The materials were handled by the two buyers and the Site Manager. Programming is my favourite part of planning. It was the dream job, but I hadn't fully recovered from my first breakdown. My nerves started jangling again, I couldn't keep still and my mind was getting faster.

Unfortunately, it coincided with the time when Diane's illness took a turn for the worse. She was in pain. Crying a lot of the time. She was crying when I went to work and still crying when I got back and it was too much for me.

In Ilkley, I had made friends with one of the buyers, Glen. At lunchtime, we used to walk down by the river and around the town. I really enjoyed the walks. I t's a nice place, Ilkley. But Glen was on a fortnight's holiday and I was on my own. One lunchtime I was walking along beside the river when I started to cry again. Great big sobs, like when I was in the church in London. I couldn't stop it. I found myself walking in a wood. The details are a bit vague here. I remember the wood, but I'm not clear about where it was. I walked back to the office, trying desperately to stop myself crying. I was late. Unfortunately, I bumped into the Managing Director. He didn't say anything, but he must have thought my behaviour was odd.

As I drove home, I was hallucinating. Swirls of colour. Strange sounds. I could hear people talking in a car that passed me. I could see the bluebells in the wood. I could hear the birds singing. How I managed to drive the car, I don't know.

THE SECOND

BREAKDOWN

Nine

I was awake all night drawing with my felt tip pens on the duvet. Diane came in to see me. We slept in separate bedrooms. I said that John Lennon was speaking to me. I said something in a Liverpool accent. I said he wanted me to take my clothes off. I can't remember much of this. I've pieced it together from what Diane told me.

In the morning, Diane rang Bootham Park and got me an appointment with a psychiatrist. I was shouting. I said I would kill the doctor if he came near me. Diane's dad took us to the hospital and her mother came too. Because I was making so much noise, they put me in the conference room. I remember a big table with lots of chairs. When the time came for me to see the psychiatrist, I wouldn't move. They fetched a wheelchair and somehow managed to get me into it. By this time I had decided to close my eyes and I kept them closed for the rest of the day. I begged them to give me a drug like the one they gave me in London to knock me out, but they didn't.

When I did eventually open my eyes, I found myself lying on a bed in a small cell where wallpaper was peeling off the wall. The door was open and a guard was stood outside. I found out later that this was the secure unit where they put patients that are a danger to the public. I wasn't there very long. Diane managed to get me out and onto Ward One.

It was the same as my first breakdown. My nerves were jangling. My mind was in turmoil. I couldn't keep still. I was shaking. During my first breakdown, I had put together several relaxation exercises, including yoga. I practised these day and night and I went jogging around the park at the front of the hospital.

Gradually my mind started to calm down. I was in hospital for 10 weeks as before. I remember the psychiatrist saying that they were surprised I had had a second breakdown, that they didn't think the first one had been that serious. They thought I had just run away to London and had a good time.

The diagnosis again was hypomania, which is a mild form of mania. They didn't mess about this time and they gave me a massive dose of Lithium 800 mgs. My psychiatrist told me that I must not go back to my job as a Planner. It was too stressful. He recommended some therapeutic work in a shop.

I started working with Oxfam for six months. And then I got a 16 hour a week job selling suitcases in a shop in McArthur, Glen. I signed on for Disabled Persons Tax Credit and got a job selling garden furniture, also at McArthur Glen. That was 20 hours a week and I did that for four years. The company got into financial difficulties and eventually went bust. It coincided with Diane's illness getting worse and she became bedbound and so I looked after her.

THE END

Also by Paul Philip Studer

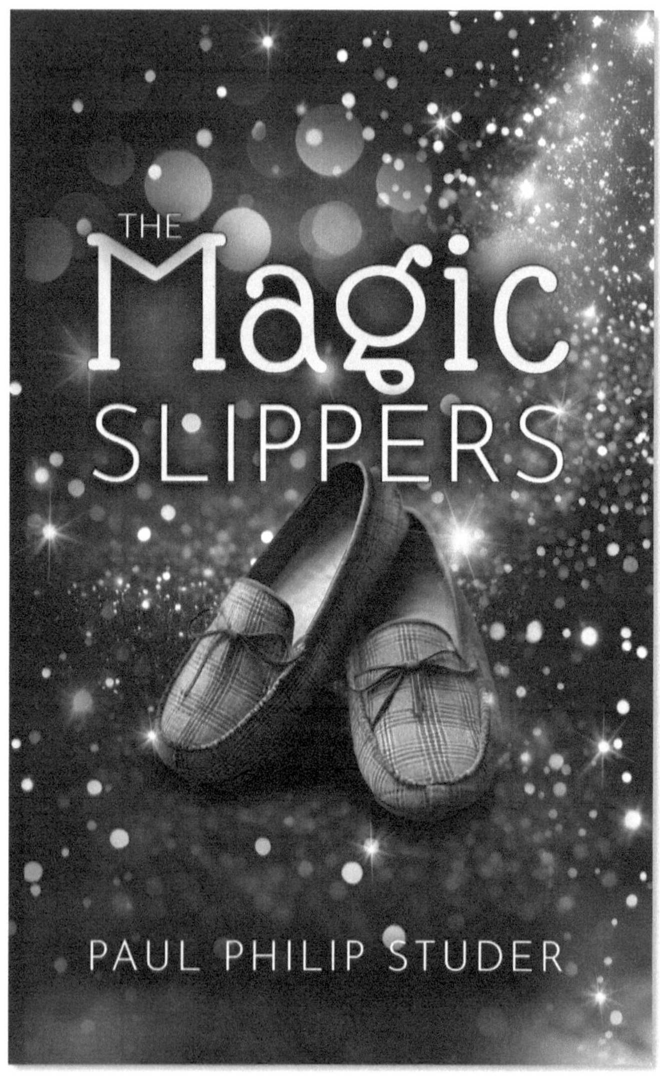

The prequel to
Escape from Moss Park Mental Hospital...

I was a casualty of my mother's ambition. My mother wanted me to do the same as my brother Anthony; he was a civil engineer.

Today was the day that the A level results would be posted on the school noticeboard.

I passed one A level: Maths - grade E. My parents went mad.

But I survived and went on to have a very good career in the building industry, as a planning surveyor.

Ironically my brother gave up his career in civil engineering and formed a company making kitchens.

The Magic Slippers

ISBN: 9781800947931

SPUG
THE MAGIC PLANET

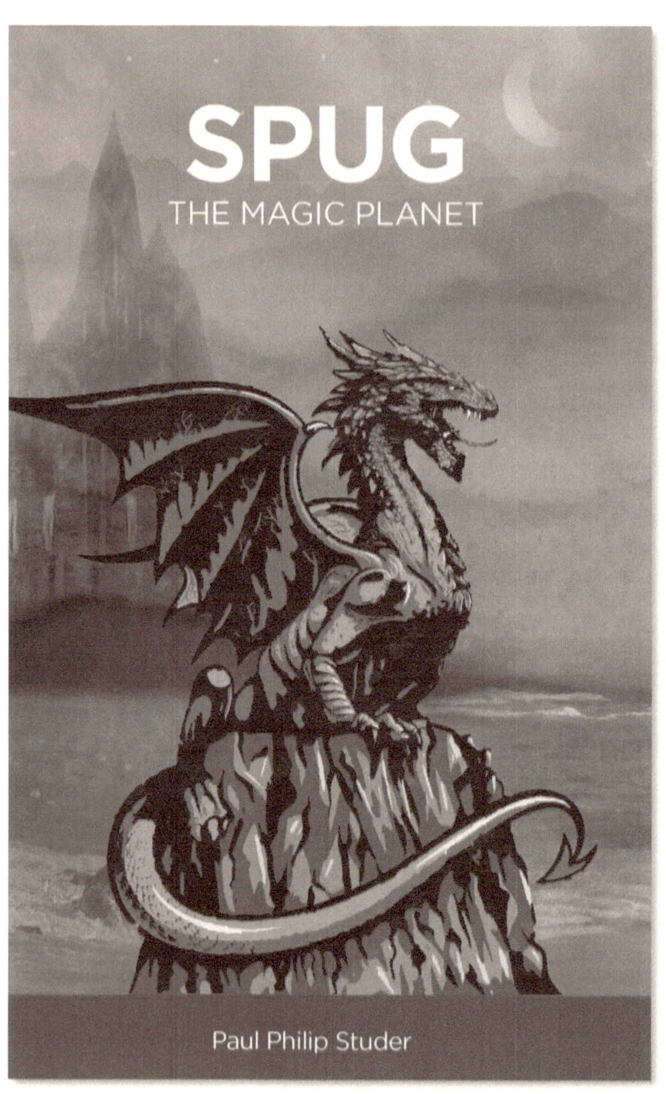

Paul Philip Studer

Tutuchamilabin or SPUG, as it is affectionately called - was a magic planet.

There were one hundred wizards who controlled its mystical lands. One of the wizards was called 'Thirty Seven', he was the Bonz's wizard. The Bonz were similar to an overgrown guinea pig, about a foot long and were governed by a King and Queen.

When the old king died, Bonz conundrums were held, to decide who should become the next King and Queen.

There was a part of SPUG where nobody ventured, on the map it said - 'There be dragons'. Wizard Zuron was determined to explore the area, when he did, he came face to face with Dragon Inferno and a tremendous battle took place.

SPUG – The Magic Planet

ISBN: 9781800947443

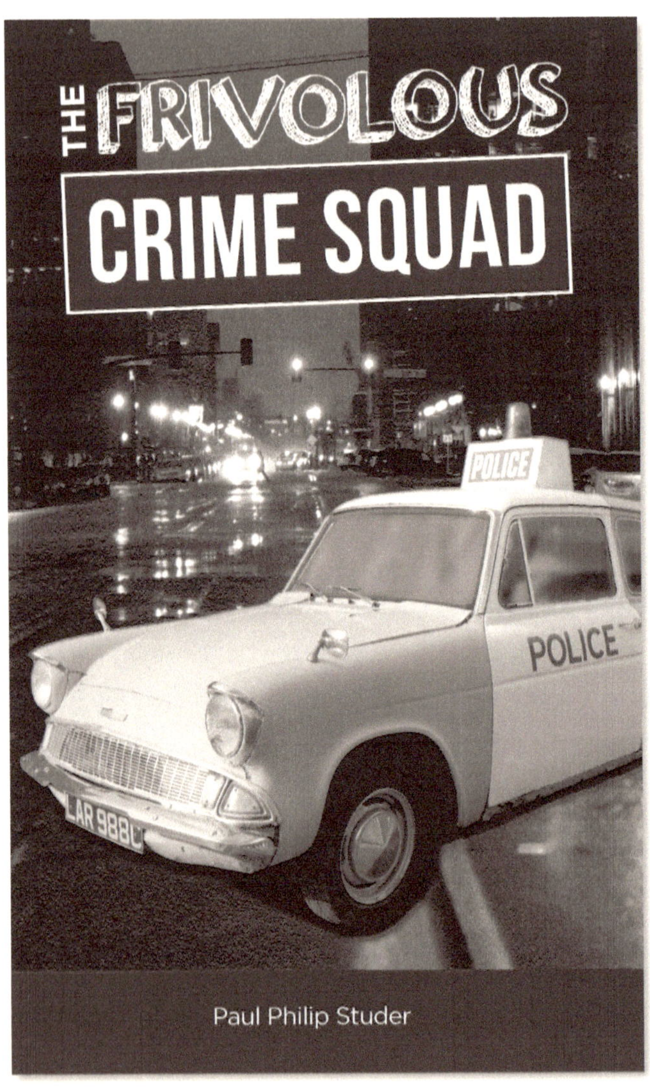

THE FRIVOLOUS
CRIME SQUAD
POLICE
POLICE
LAR 988L
Paul Philip Studer

It has always struck me as odd to have a police unit called The Serious Crime Squad. All crime is serious by definition. I know what they mean by 'Serious Crime: murder, rape, bank robbery, for example. 'Serious' is defined as:

1. Demanding or characterised by careful consideration or application.
2. Acting or speaking sincerely and in earnest, rather than in a joking or half-hearted manner.

You could apply that definition to investigating any crime. So, I have flipped it on its head - the opposite of serious is 'frivolous'. 'Frivolous' is defined as:
Not having any serious purpose or value.

I have invented crimes that the Serious Crime Squad would not touch:

1. Stealing collection money from a church.
2. Wheelie bin fire.
3. Theft of five pairs of very expensive knickers.

It follows therefore, that these crimes are frivolous; hence the name of the book!

The Frivolous Crime Squad

ISBN: 9781800947627

THE ADVENTURES
OF VINNY

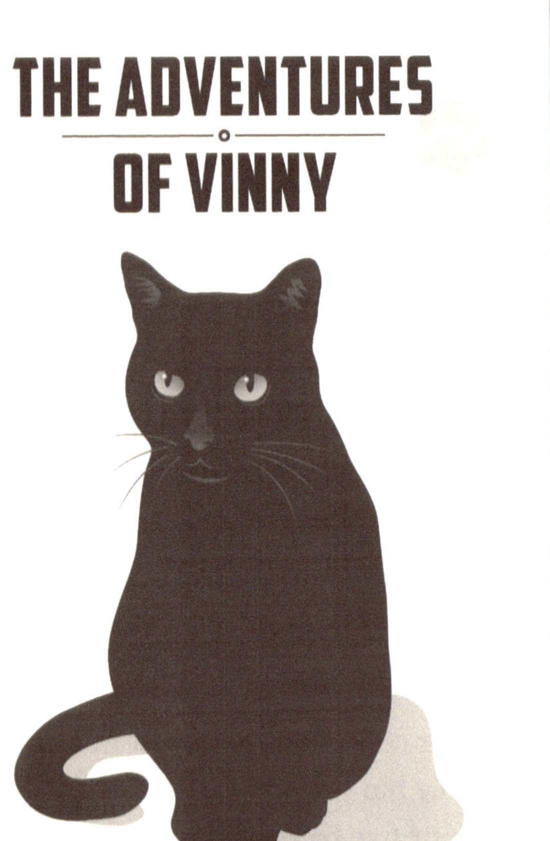

Paul Philip Studer

Vinny was a very streetwise cat - but one day, he forgot himself and caused the most horrendous car crash, involving multiple vehicles.

In the aftermath, the local Policeman - Sergeant Ventress, wants to have Vinny put to sleep, to ensure that he doesn't cause any further catastrophies. Unfortunately, no-one will tell the Sergeant where Vinny lives (they all know, but remain tight lipped)!

Other adventures include a very unpleasant journey to Whitby, spent under the bonnet of Elvis's delivery van. Another time, Vinny ends up in Aberdeen, stowed away in a removal van.

The Adventures of Vinny

ISBN: 9781800947924